Seeds
OF
Hope

A JOURNEY THROUGH
MEDICATION AND MADNESS
TOWARD MEANING

JOCELYN PEDERSEN

Moonglade Press
Publishing New Works by Uncommon Voices
Distributed by IngramSpark
www.moongladepress.com

ISBN: 978-0-9987639-5-8
Library of Congress Control Number: 2019919314

Printed in the U.S.A.

This book is dedicated to my God who gave me life,
my husband and children who make it a life worth living,
and my mystic friend Marjorie, whose vision
and persistence helped me reveal the beauty
of such a life within its pages.

Contents

Preface

This story is about the journey we all make through the dark waters of life's most unexpected and seemingly insurmountable adversities. It's about the seeds of hope we plant in soils of faith when the sun is shining, and the weather is calm. They are seeds that can only truly take root when the rains descend, and turbulent waters rise. Fragile tendrils of hope grow until, one day, they finally touch the sunlight as it breaks through the clouds to illuminate the fruits of our ascent.

As a woman and a follower of The Church of Jesus Christ of Latter-day Saints (Mormon) I want to present my view on hope and healing. I do not speak for The Church of Jesus Christ. I am not anti-psychiatry nor do I seek to offer medical advice. I am an expert on my own experience. What I offer in this book are hope and understanding.

JOCELYN PEDERSEN

Prologue

Members of The Church of Jesus Christ of Latter-day Saints have a very different view of Eve than most Christians. We see her as one of the most courageous human beings in all of creation. She lived in a place where everything was ideal. There was no death, no sadness, no hunger or loneliness. Everything existed as it was when first created, uncorrupted, unchanging, eternal. While God warned Adam and Eve about partaking of the fruit of the tree of knowledge of good and evil, it was a choice, an opportunity designed to allow his children to either remain as they were or to become like Him. But, since becoming like God meant change, Adam and Eve had to transgress a law so they could become corruptible.

Whether in mortality or in the eternal realm, there are laws that cannot be circumvented. Like the law of gravity, one may choose to jump off a cliff, but one cannot choose whether or not to fall towards the center of the earth. Gravity will have her say whether or not we chose to listen. So it was with Eve in the garden. She could have chosen to remain where she was and stay the same, or she could choose to jump, embracing all the consequences that came with it. I imagine she didn't know what it was like to fall, but she knew there would be pain and death. And while the serpent beguiled her with soft denials of the fruits of such a choice, Eve acted on her desire to create. The need to fulfill her purpose as a daughter, wife, and mother outweighed any desire for comfort she may have had. Eve chose to consume knowledge and everything that comes with it. Our mother helped her husband to see that falling was the only way to become who they were meant to be, so together, they lept.

We all did.

CHAPTER 1
Connecting the Dots

You can't connect the dots looking forward; you can only connect them looking backwards. So you have to trust that the dots will somehow connect in your future. You have to trust in something — your gut, destiny, life, karma, whatever.

STEVE JOBS, AUGUST 25, 2011

Little did I know how right Mr. Jobs was when he made that statement in 2011. I had no idea at the time that my decisions to take a series of medications prescribed to me by a trusted friend and family doctor would lead me to write this book, co-found a nonprofit, and lecture to mental health professionals all over the world on a subject about which I knew very little in 2011. I didn't know ten years earlier, in 2001, while I was preparing to graduate summa cum laude from Brigham Young University, that the young man who kept "accidentally" running into me on my way to and from campus would become not just the love of my life but someone whom I would rely on for my very existence. A man who would prove to be the hero of my life's story, a story I never intended to tell.

It never occurred to me that our "chance encounters" were orchestrated. Paul would watch for me from his window, and as I was walking downhill from campus, he would manage to look like he was just on his way up. Six-foot-one and of Danish descent, Paul looked like a baby-faced Viking. Not at all the type I was used to. I had spent much of my time at BYU surrounded by Native American, Polynesian, and Latin American dancers from Living Legends, the ethnic dance team I auditioned for my sophomore year. These are the people I danced with, lived with, traveled with, and who became my family. Not that I didn't date young men from a variety of backgrounds when I had any time outside of dancing and my studies. It's just that growing up Hispanic, in a predominantly Latin/Italian community, I was used to a certain type. Paul was very unlike the caramel-toned guys who normally caught my eye, but I had apparently caught his.

Being at a school established by The Church of Jesus Christ of Latter-day Saints means that every student who is a member of the church is assigned a congregation (ward) to attend based on location. That semester I had moved into an apartment that put me in Paul's ward. He told me the first time he noticed me was when I stood up to bear my testimony in a fast and testimony sacrament meeting[1] at church. It was the beginning of the semester, and I didn't know anyone in the ward yet, so I didn't notice Paul when he came up to talk to me after that sacrament meeting.

"That's because there was a whole bunch of other guys surrounding you after the meeting," Paul told me a few years later. "I couldn't

---

1   Every first Sunday of the month we fast for two meals and give the money we would have spent on food to the poor. Then, after taking the sacrament, we have an open mic where anybody can come up to the pulpit and share whatever they feel prompted by the spirit to say about God's plan of salvation and their own faith-building experiences. Testimonies aren't written down or prepared ahead of time.

get past them to say hi! I guess they were as impressed by you as I was."

"Are you telling me a bunch of guys were flirting with me because my testimony was so awesome?" I joked back.

"Well, I don't remember what you said exactly, but I remember it was powerful and thinking, 'wow, if that girl would marry me, that's the kind of girl I would marry right now.'"

I tried to remember what I had said. I remember I had spoken about how much I loved the gospel, and how on fire I was to constantly share my testimony of it with others throughout high school. I explained that I grew up in a place where very few people had ever heard of The Church, which gave me lots of opportunities to share the gospel. And yet I'd had more experiences at BYU with sharing the gospel than ever. It doesn't really translate into writing, but I remember feeling the holy spirit strongly as I spoke.

That's just how I was back then. I had a fire of faith that burned so bright; it often blinded me to any darkness around me. I assumed that flame would always burn brighter than the darkness. Little did I know when I stood up in church that day that I was capable of enduring pain so deep it could hollow me out, expand the boundaries of my soul, and leave behind a vacuum so powerful I would be forced to fill it with either darkness or light. I was faced with just such a decision in North Carolina three years after Paul heard me bear that testimony.

Everything was going as planned. Graduate college, check. Marry a returned missionary in the temple, check. Have a baby and then have three or four more, not too far apart, but not too close together. Check. It was a good plan. Paul and I were sealed for time and eternity in the Salt Lake City Temple on August 10, 2001. I had graduated earlier that spring and was able to support him through his last year and a half of schooling. When we moved to North Carolina in 2003, after his graduation, we decided it would be a good time to start our family. I figured we'd get pregnant quickly since I wasn't taking the pill, a decision I made after turning into an unreasonable, sobbing, angry, bloated mess on birth control within the first few months of being married. A girlfriend saved my relationship with my husband by recommending a book called *Taking Charge of Your Fertility*. It was all about a natural method of birth control, and it had worked beautifully for the last two years. Since we weren't in the habit of using contraceptives anyway, Paul and I decided just to let nature take its course.

To be honest, nature took a little longer than I expected; I assumed I'd get pregnant right away. I have a tendency to live in the moment, so a few months later, when I couldn't figure out why my nerves at my new teaching position hadn't gone away yet, pregnancy wasn't really on my mind. I'd already been working at the school for a month, and I still had to run to the bathroom every morning with what I thought were loose bowels from a nervous stomach. It was something I'd experienced frequently as a performer. The idea that my bathroom trips might be a symptom of something else never even crossed my mind until I complained about them to my co-worker, Saisha. "Well if you're not sick maybe you're pregnant," my friend said in her matter of fact, southern way. My eyes grew wider and wider while Saisha laughed harder and harder as I slowly came to the realization that she had just hit the nail directly on the head.

I broke the news to Paul by showing him my positive test result the next morning. We had never been happier. But I was afraid to give myself completely over to my joy, afraid that I might get too attached to someone who wasn't even born yet, only to be disappointed if something went wrong later on. It wasn't like me to be so fearful, but I couldn't shake the feeling, so I called my mom for reassurance. "Jocelyn, you don't need to worry," she assured me. "The women in our family have fast deliveries and healthy babies. You came so fast they didn't even have time to give me an epidural! You'll be ok." I felt better after our conversation. Everything would be ok.

I let my fear give way to love and enjoyed every moment of being pregnant. I blasted the baby's favorite music in the car as I drove down the freeway. I loved feeling him dance to Josh Groban in my belly. Every night, Paul and I would use our store-bought monitor to listen to Ethan's heartbeat. It was never hard to find. We'd play a game of poke, where one of us would poke my tummy, and Ethan would poke back. When we had our 24-week ultrasound, our son showed us how truly aware he was of what was going on around him. We eagerly watched his image on the black and white screen next to the exam table on which I was lying. As the probe glided across my belly, Ethan followed it exactly with his index finger. His head moved in unison almost as if he could see us with his unopened eyes. The technician marveled and said it was the most incredible thing he'd ever seen. I knew Ethan was special.

One afternoon, as I prepared his nursery, I heard the next show announced on the TV. They would be doing a special on caring for newborn infants. I perked up and listened as the guest spoke about the five S's, side, suck, swaddle, sway, and shhh. I took a mental note, so I would know how to swaddle Ethan properly when he arrived. As I did so, a thought entered into my mind, almost like a voice that wasn't mine, saying, "That will never happen." "What a terrible thing to say!" I thought. But the feeling was so overpowering that I ran into the next room and frantically pulled out the images of Ethan's ultrasound. I stared at them as if to prove to myself that he was real, that this hadn't all been just a lovely dream. Surely this was just my old worries creeping back in. I pushed that experience to the back of my mind and went on with my life as though nothing had happened.

Perhaps, if I'd been more astute, I would have realized the conversations I was having with my son in my dreams were not merely those "crazy pregnancy" dreams my friends and family had warned me about, but were actually my spirit interacting with that of a fully formed soul. Although his little body had not finished growing, Ethan's spirit, like everyone's, is already as old as eternity. I came to know later on from various scriptures and my own experience that while in the womb, a baby is not necessarily bound by the same limitations of mortality that we are. Our nighttime conversations made more sense to me with this knowledge, even if it was only in hindsight.

In my dreams, my son would be born too early. I was horrified to find myself alone in my apartment, holding the perfectly formed body of a baby that was too small to survive more than a few minutes.

"Please," I pleaded, "please go back in."

"It's time," Ethan would reply.

"No! It's too early, I need you to stay in a little longer, just a little longer, and then you can come out."

"I need to come out now," was his response.

Terrified, I went on:

"Please, no, please, stay with me!" I repeated over and over as he inched closer and closer to death.

The dream always ended there. The terror I felt upon waking would dissolve into relief as I realized that I had not miscarried. The baby was still alive. I kept all these things to myself and enjoyed my blissful, if willful, ignorance. Looking back now, I believe Ethan held on for me. He was my son, and he did what I asked, even though what I required of him may have been painful.

It was cold in the early morning of December 17th, 2003, as my friend Oni pulled up to our apartment with her little boy. Oni and I wanted to be first to arrive at the department store for a big sale that was going on, so we could have our pick of the baby clothes. I'd been up late the night before. Paul and I were having a hard time finding Ethan's heartbeat. Instead of his normally playful kicks and punches, I felt something more rhythmic and jerking inside me. Maybe these were the hiccups everyone said babies get that I had never felt before with mine. I became increasingly worried as I squeezed my nine-month girth between the racks of little onesies. My baby was too still. I could tell he wasn't moving. I asked Oni if she would drive me to the doctor's office.

"I'm sorry. This baby doesn't have a heartbeat," the doctor quietly announced.

"What? What does that mean? Do something! Perform an emergency C-section! Give me a solution, something, ANYTHING!"

I yelled the words in my mind as I stared quietly at the perfectly still baby on the black and white screen above my bed. I stared hard at the image as if to prove to myself that this was real, that it wasn't all just a terrible dream. After the doctor left the room Oni, who had been at my side, asked, "What do you need me to do for you?" I choked back the tears as I responded, "Will you kneel with me to pray?" That was the last prayer I would utter for some time.

It wasn't that I had lost faith in God. In fact, I knew now more than ever how aware he had been of my baby boy and me. I couldn't be mad at him. He had tried to prepare me, and not just that afternoon in front of the TV. There were words spoken in the priesthood blessing[2] Paul had given me a few weeks earlier which, though confusing at the time, now all made sense. There were lines in the patriarchal blessing[3] I had received when I was 16 years old that talked about understanding what it must have felt like for my Heavenly Father to give up his only begotten son. I knew God was real, and I knew he had let this happen. I felt both loved and betrayed by him. I'd been hurt many times in my life by people I cared about. I'd been abused (another story for another time), bullied, and beaten. But never had anyone hurt me so deeply as the one being I trusted most in all the universe hurt me on that day.

After kneeling to pray with me, Oni called her husband, Chien, who was working with Paul. Oni explained everything that was going on to them. About a half-hour later, Paul and Chien arrived at the hospital. I asked them to give me a priesthood blessing. I didn't realize at the time how unfair it was to require that of my bereaved husband. As he and Chien lay their hands on my head, the words of comfort I expected from my Heavenly Father didn't come out of Paul's mouth. Instead, he uttered something about how natural things just happen in this world, and we have to learn to accept that. "Wait; what?" I thought, "wasn't this all supposed to be a part of God's plan? Isn't

---

2   In a priesthood blessing a servant of the Lord exercises the priesthood, as moved upon by the Holy Ghost, to call upon the powers of heaven for the benefit of the person being blessed. Such blessings are conferred by holders of the Melchizedek Priesthood, which has the keys of all the spiritual blessings of the Church... Priesthood Blessings: churchofjesuschrist.org

3   Patriarchal blessings can only be given by an ordained patriarch whose sole calling is to confer these blessings. "Patriarchal blessings include a declaration of a person's lineage in the house of Israel and contain personal counsel from the Lord." Patriarchal Blessings, churchofjesuschrist.org

there supposed to be some greater meaning to all of this?" I didn't think it was possible to be more crushed than I already was. Now I realize the words my husband spoke were more about his despair than my sorrow. But at the time, they were powerful enough to extinguish the little spark of hope I still had in the midst of that dimly lit ultrasound room.

We consulted with the doctor after that about our options. He wanted us to wait until the baby came naturally and then deliver him. But the longer I waited, the more Ethan's body would deteriorate as it decomposed in my womb. That wasn't a thought I could bear. I pleaded with the OBGYN to deliver him as soon as possible. He told us to come back in a few hours, and he would induce labor. My parents were frantically trying to get a flight from Utah to North Carolina, but there was no way they could possibly make it in time for the delivery. When we returned to the hospital, we were surprised to see Dottie, a woman from our ward in Mooresville, waiting for us in the lobby. She walked over to us and held out a shaking hand. In her palm was a small, disposable camera. She was crying. Dottie told us about the stillbirth of her first baby boy. "Take pictures of your baby," she instructed. "You're going to want to see them when he's gone. And don't let the nurses take him away until you're ready. Spend as much time with him as you can. They're some of the only memories you'll have." She hugged us and sent us on our way up to labor and delivery.

When we arrived, it was as if Paul and I were a pair of lepers. Nobody wanted to be in the room with us. The nurses turned invisible, even when we called for them. The doctor went home, despite my protests that women in my family tend to deliver babies quickly. He insisted it was my first and that I wouldn't progress until morning.

The only person who wasn't afraid to stay with us was a receptionist working at the front desk. Dede had found out about our situation and came by to offer us some comfort. She left while they inserted one fourth of a Pitocin pill to start my labor. She returned with a gray, baby-sized teddy bear which she placed in my arms. "Here, sweetie, it helps to have something to hold in your arms that feels like a baby." For the first time since entering the hospital, I overcame my shock and suddenly burst into tears. "Oh, I'm sorry. I'm so sorry. I didn't mean to make you cry!" But I didn't want Dede to feel bad. I was so grateful to her for being my angel. I wasn't crying about the teddy bear or my baby. I was crying because I felt so pathetic and helpless.

When I started having back to back contractions, the nurses flushed the Pitocin and called the doctor. He was too far away. I was already dilated to a seven by the time the anesthesiologist arrived. She kept running in and out of the room, calling the doctor and asking for directions on how to proceed. Meanwhile, I felt like something was on fire in between my legs. I cried out for Dede. "What is that?" I whimpered. "Oh baby, that's you tearing down there because you're coming so fast." The anesthesiologist asked me to curve my back and stay as still as I could so she could insert the epidural. I tried to do what she asked, but my back was contracting so hard it didn't take. She gave me a second dose, and still, there was no relief from the pain. By the time the doctor made it back to the hospital, I was dilated to nine, and Ethan's head was crowning. He insisted the anesthesiologist give me another epidural then he put something in my IV to knock me out. He gave Paul something to knock him out too. We were both out of our minds with grief. We didn't realize how odd it all was. It didn't cross my mind that the physician never intended to deliver our baby and was doing everything he could to avoid delivering Ethan. Even in hindsight, it makes no sense to me, but that's what happened. My baby and I stayed like that, suspended in the last stage of labor for seven and a half hours until my other doctor came the next morning to deliver us. Left to ourselves we kissed and stroked our sons lifeless, now mutilated, and torn body. Then Paul dutifully took pictures as Dottie instructed. We finally handed him over to the nurses and went home. I kneeled beside my bed that night and tried to say a prayer, but no words came out. I was too heartbroken. I knew God knew this. I knew he wasn't angry with me and that when I was ready to speak with him again, he would be there to receive me with open arms. I was at peace with God, but I didn't feel like talking to him.

After the funeral, my mother stayed to help pack up the baby things and get me back on my feet. Before she left for the airport, mom insisted I needed sleep and offered me some Ambien. I told her that, despite everything, I was sleeping just fine. She insisted anyway. I knew she didn't want to leave me alone with my grief. It was one of the only things she felt she could do for me. I tried the Ambien. I woke up the next morning unable to move, feeling like someone was standing in the room next to me. Was that Ethan touching my hair? After spending the second morning on Ambien attempting to swat an imaginary fly from my face with leaden arms, I decided enough was enough. I never told my mom about my reaction to the Ambien or my decision to chuck the extra pills she'd left behind in the trash.

I didn't give it much thought at the time, but what I had experienced was a symptom known as sleep paralysis. It wasn't until years later that I realized there was something significant about my reaction to those two little white pills.

CHAPTER 2

Dividing the Light from the Darkness

The most important step a man can take. It's not the first one, is it?
It's the next one. Always the next step...

BRANDON SANDERSON, OATHBRINGER

It was almost a year after Ethan's death before I could really be myself again and look people in the eye without feeling like I had somehow forgotten to wear pants that day. Despite my embarrassment at being so exposed by the rawness of my feelings, I experienced profound peace the summer after his passing. It came after countless prayers and pleas with my Heavenly Father to let me see my son again. I wanted an experience like those I'd read about in the books people gave me written by other members of the church who'd lost their babies. One story spoke about a mother whose son visited her after he passed away. He told her to let go of her grieving so he could move on and do the work the Lord had for him on the other side of the veil. Oh, how I wanted to see my son again too! My greatest sorrow came from never being able to look him in the eyes, whisper goodbye into his little ear and know that he felt my parting kiss on his soft cheek. I guess what I needed is what others call closure. I scoured the scriptures for angelic encounters and evidence of babies who were spiritually aware in the womb.

A few months after the funeral, Paul and I drove the two hours it takes to get from where we lived to the new temple [1] in Columbia, South Carolina. I sat in the car with a burning question on my mind, aside from my desire to see Ethan. It was a question posed to me by a friend going through a crisis of faith. As I worked through the endowment session, pondering what answer I could give her, my eyes were suddenly opened, and I understood things I never had before about the temple ceremony.It was as if I saw myself go through the entire plan of salvation, from the premortal life into mortality and after the first resurrection when the righteous will live during the reign of Christ on the earth. I saw myself standing next to my son, in a resurrected immortal body, while he, resurrected with the promise of a full life in a mortal state and raised to adulthood by loving parents, worked with me and others to seal the entire family of our Heavenly Mother and Father together. Afterward, I couldn't wait to meet Paul in the celestial room and tell him what I had learned.

As we sat in that reverent atmosphere, I related what had been revealed to me. As I did, I felt a familiar feeling. It was similar to something I'd felt when I was 16 years old, except not nearly so powerful. Instead of a flame of fire that consumed me from head to toe, this was more like a tingly light in the center of my soul. I knew what it was, though, and I knew it was God's way of telling me what I was saying was true. I wished that feeling would reach out like a tongue of fire and touch Paul as it had my friend to whom I had been bearing my

1   "Members of The Church of Jesus Christ of Latter-day Saints follow the biblical practice of worshipping in temples. They believe temples are places of special sacredness where they can make binding promises with God and feel closer to Him... "What is the Purpose of Temples of the Church of Jesus Christ of Latter-day Saints? Comeuntochrist.org

testimony when I felt consumed by the spirit, an undeniable witness that he couldn't dismiss. But Paul would have to find the answer to his sorrows in his own way, many years later. For me, it was enough. I didn't get the chance to say goodbye, but I did see my son again in my own way. What's more, I knew that I would see him again one day and raise him to adulthood in a more perfect world. It was a glorious branch of hope that lifted me out of deep pools of tears, as I learned to live without my son month after month and year after year.

Though the waters were sometimes bitter, they had no power to make me sink into despair. No power that is, until the bitter pools erupted, swelling until they formed an endless sea of misery. Misery, it turns out, can be purchased at your local pharmacy. The next time I took Ambien, it was given to me by my OBGYN in Orem, Utah. The summer after Ethan's passing, we left North Carolina for Utah. But we couldn't leave our son behind. So, after exhuming Ethan from his unmarked grave, Paul carefully placed his little casket in the back of our U-Haul, and we began our journey back to a place where we could be closer to family. Like the pioneers, we carried our son west with us across the plains. We buried him again, this time beneath the shadow of the Rocky Mountains.

I was in my second year of teaching at a Title I school, not 15 minutes from where Paul and I had first met, when I became pregnant with our second baby boy. I was considered high risk after what happened with our first. My OBGYN was very cautious but also optimistic. Dr. Elder was a numbers man. He liked to give me statistics on all the variables that could lead to our bringing this baby home safe and sound. I liked that part of our relationship. The part I didn't like was when he would try to use his stats to convince me I needed medication. He offered me drugs for morning sickness, constipation, cramps, anything, and everything. I always declined them. Growing up with a chiropractor for a father gave me a healthy distrust of the medical profession and besides, I was fine.

It wasn't until I came down with what was diagnosed as a 'rip roarin' bladder infection that I became worried. The infection started preterm labor, and with each contraction, Nathaniel's heart rate would dip dangerously low. We discovered that just like Ethan, Nathaniel had the cord wrapped tightly around his neck. The contractions were strangling my baby. Dr. Elder was determined not to let me lose two babies. He had me monitored 24/7 in the hospital on bed rest.

With Paul at work all day and very few friends able to visit, I was alone most of the time, staring at the monitor, waiting with bated breath each time Nathaniel's heart slowed down for it to return to normal. Dr. Elder practically tried to force-feed me antidepressants in the hospital. But I put my foot down. Finally, after the umpteenth night of lying awake in anticipation of my nurse coming into my room in the middle of the night to adjust my belly monitor and check my blood pressure, I acquiesced to Dr. Elder's pleas for me to get some more sleep. "Besides," he argued, "Studies have shown Ambien doesn't cross the placenta. The baby won't be affected by it." Convinced, I took Ambien for the second time in my life, only this time, it wasn't for a couple of days, it was for a couple of months.

Nathaniel was delivered six weeks early by emergency C-section and, despite the unexplained bruising all along the right side of his face and body, was declared perfectly healthy and sent home a few days later. Dr. Elder proudly proclaimed it was the steroid shots he had given us that prepared Nathaniel's lungs for an early birth and which made a stay in the neonatal intensive care unit unnecessary. I went home happy but feeling very unprepared. I hadn't been able to read any of the books I'd planned to on nursing or caring for a newborn, despite lying around all day long in a hospital bed. My eyes just wouldn't focus, and there was this thick cloud that blanketed my brain the entire time I was on bed rest. I figured it had something to do with the magnesium sulfate coursing through my veins via the IV drip. In reality, these were symptoms of an adverse reaction to Ambien.

When we got home, I stopped the sleeping pills. It was my first real cold turkey.[2] Adjusting to sleeping without the medication plus the new baby made the next couple of sleepless months seem totally normal. I didn't realize how abnormal I was feeling or how difficult it was for me to make reasonable decisions during those first few months. I would berate Paul for not getting home exactly on time and leaving me with a crying baby all day. I freaked out that my son was not getting all the nutrition he needed from breastfeeding. I couldn't ever seem to just sit down and enjoy the miracle of holding a living, breathing baby boy in my arms.

Despite my irrational behavior, I knew something really was wrong with Nathaniel. My baby never slept more than 45 minutes at a stretch. He was frantic all the time. He couldn't keep down food or pass bowel movements on his own. He seemed like he was in pain, and there was little I could do to help him. Paul and I used the 5 S's with some success. In fact, we used the technique religiously day and night, all night long sometimes it seemed. Paul confided in me that he

---

2   The sudden, abrupt cessation of medication

got so aggressive with the shooshing and shaking some nights he was worried he might, in his sleep-deprived state, end up hurting his son.

"He's just colicky," was our only reply from the doctors. But this went way beyond a newborn baby struggling to adjust to life outside the womb. My family still jokes about how calm all the other babies in the hospital nursery were, whereas Nathaniel flopped around so violently they thought he might flip right out of the baby cot! How was I to know the combination of Ambien and steroids Nathaniel was exposed to in the womb were a toxic elixir that would lead to a lifetime of problems? Nathaniel wasn't colicky. He was going through withdrawal.

Even though I was ignorant as to the source of our troubles, I was given the gift of knowledge in other ways. A friend from church, a mother of many adopted special needs children, helped me find a craniosacral therapist who got Nathaniel to start sleeping five hours at night. It was a miracle! Another friend introduced us to her mother, a zone balancing practitioner who showed me how to stimulate Nathaniel's colon. At four-months-old, he passed a bowel movement on his own for the first time after she worked on him. Another miracle! After that, all skepticism flew out the window. I began to study everything I could about alternative therapies, nutrition, and supplementation. Life got better. I got better, Nathaniel got better, even Paul got better!

Nathaniel still definitely had some sensitivities, but the strict diet I created for him managed things well, and besides, the doctors had been no help. Over the years, we did allergy testing, a swallow study, and various other tests, all of which told us nothing. I relied on my intuition and my faith in God. He'd miraculously healed me as a baby from toxic epidural necrolysis. He healed my sorrow when I had no baby of my own to cradle in my arms. Now, I was certain, God would take care of my son.

CHAPTER 3

Falling

When the darkness of night falls, we do not despair and worry that the sun is extinguished. We do not postulate that the sun is not there or is dead. We understand that we are in a shadow, that the earth will continue to rotate, and that eventually the rays of the sun will reach us once again.

DIETER F. UCHTDORF, SEPTEMBER 30, 2017

Ok, God, that's it. I'm fed up with you not upholding your end of the bargain. I've been doing my part; I'm just asking for a little help here, and I'm not getting it! I had faith. But it wasn't rewarded. I guess I'm just going to have to do this on my own, and if I'm going to do it by myself, then I need some sleep. Bye

This was a very different kind of prayer for me. In my defense, I was sleep-deprived. It was 2010, and over the past month, I'd had two children in the hospital, and a husband whose occupation as a builder during the housing market crash became practically nonexistent. The money didn't stress me out. My family history was filled with stories of parents and grandparents who'd worked their way out of poverty to live a good life. I saw financial struggle as a rite of passage. My parents were poor when I was little. There was no indignity to it. In fact, these were the experiences that led to some of the greatest faith-building stories in my family, the tales which nurtured my testimony from the time I was young.

No, what really shook my foundation was the insomnia. Sleep was my Achilles heel. Even in college, I could handle any sort of roommate, except for the ones who messed with my sleep. They could be smelly, loud, obnoxious, and I would just brush it off. But if they ruined my sleep ... well, that was just unforgivable. This was kind of my attitude towards God that day as I rose from my knees. I couldn't forgive him for making me go without sleep. Without sleep, the weeks, months, and years of trials were suddenly magnified, like light through a glass. The lens of insomnia intensified and focused everything to one burning point, the heat of which burned my altar of faith down to a little nub. Why, when I had been doing everything so right, was everything going so wrong?

I had stood by Paul when he lost his job and was patient with him as he struggled with his own personal demons, now exacerbated by his unemployment. To help support the family, I worked nights while pregnant with Lucy so I could still be home during the day to care for our three-year-old son. I never complained when we had to gut the house and hawk everything that would fetch a decent price. I served enthusiastically in my callings at church as a teacher and a pianist. I made do when we had no car and found ways to keep Nathaniel entertained in our little split-level home. Heck, I even managed to deliver Lucy outside of a hospital! Of course, that wasn't about money.

You see, God and I had an understanding. Just a year before my bout of insomnia, right before Lucy was conceived, I knelt in my living room to say another rare kind of prayer. It was a covenant I felt I needed to make between myself and God.

Dear Heavenly Father, I think I'm ready to have another baby, and I believe this is thy will too. If it is thy will for me to bring another one of thy children into this world, then I can't go through the same experiences again. After what happened with Ethan and Nathaniel I can't do this in a hospital. I just don't trust doctors anymore. I don't want to be surrounded by the people who hurt me, dismissed me, and let my first baby die. I can't go through months of drugs and bed rest like I did with Nathaniel, alone day and night, worrying he might die at any minute and then have him by C-section, coming out all bruised, looking like Ethan did. I have to do this naturally. I want to use a midwife. I NEED to do this outside of a hospital. Please. I've been working so hard to heal my body with the foods and methods I've been studying. I feel stronger and healthier than ever. I'm ready. I come before thee humbly now to make this covenant. I promise to raise the child thou sendest us unto thee, in righteousness in love and in health. If thou wilt bless me with a natural pregnancy and safe delivery, I promise to teach this baby thy word, to help her develop her talents and prepare her to be an instrument in thy hands for good. Please hear my words. Make this covenant with me. I pray in the name of Jesus Christ, Amen.

I stood up. I felt peace. I knew I was going to have this baby naturally. I knew it was going to be a girl, and I knew her name would be Lucy. I was confident everything would be ok. Even when Dr. Elder berated me at my next appointment, and threatened me by saying he had already made sure no one at his clinic would touch me if I chose to have this baby naturally, even when he stormed out of the room leaving me half naked on the exam table with the door open, I felt at peace.

Trusting that my midwife, a master herbalist, could get my baby and me safely through a VBAC,[1] I had little fear when a few waves rocked the boat. There were some symptoms which could have been signs of a much bigger problem, but they were actually caused by a benign polyp. No big deal. Overly cautious about a bladder infection creating similar problems during this pregnancy as with my second, our family doctor regularly prescribed me antibiotics at the slightest sign of a urinary tract infection. It seemed like I tested positive every month for one of those. I didn't love the idea of taking antibiotics, especially after all the work I'd put into healing my gut, but I dutifully took my prescriptions as prescribed. Despite all that, I was full of positive energy, happy to play with my son during the day, prepare a meal ahead of time for him and Paul, and then go to work in the late afternoon or evening until closing. Sometimes we had to get creative about transportation and rely on neighbors for babysitting until Paul could get home, but Nathaniel was happy, and that was all that mattered to me.

After Lucy was born, I made sure never to ask Paul to get up with her in the middle of the night, as he had with Nathaniel when the baby and I were in withdrawal. When Lucy went into the ER with meningitis, and Paul was out of town, I took care of everything. When he met us at the hospital, I volunteered to be the one to stay

---

1   vaginal birth after cesarean

with her all night and day so he could continue to look for work and so I could breastfeed my sick baby. I didn't complain about the impossibility of sleeping in the inadequate reclining chair the hospital provided. I spent those weeks of sleepless nights praying for my baby girl. I asked others to fast and pray for her. I had every confidence God would protect the child he had helped to bring so miraculously into the world.

I'd done everything I could to prove myself to God and my husband. I even forced myself to stay awake after Lucy and I got home from Primary Children's Hospital because I felt bad about Paul spending yet another sleepless night with Nathaniel. This time, it was our son's turn to end up in the ER. Nathaniel had barely finished potty training before Lucy got sick. Unfortunately, he wasn't comfortable telling grandma and grandpa when he needed to use the bathroom, and we didn't realize until he got home that he hadn't done so in weeks. Twice in one month, he went to the ER with impacted bowels, and each time I feared it was going to break my husband. Too many hospitals, too many reminders of what we had lost, and might have lost. Paul's heart hadn't healed as mine had since Ethan's death. I felt like I needed to protect him. It was my job now to worry. Paul was the one who always worried, and I wanted to relieve his burden. I would do the worrying for him. If it was a competition as to who would have the most sleepless nights, I would win. If Paul had to listen to his son's screams in the middle of the night, alone in the ER, then I would keep vigil until he returned. Every time my eyelids drooped, and I felt the warm stupor of sleep wash over me, I would jerk myself awake. Nobody could accuse me of not doing my part.

After Paul and Nathaniel got home from their second ER visit, and everything settled down, I gave myself permission to go to sleep. I laid my head on my pillow, waiting for that warm floaty feeling to take over. It was something I had conditioned my mind and body to do during hypnobirthing.[2] In fact, all I had to do to sink into a deep slumber was play through the peaceful, wonderful labor I had with Lucy in my mind. That's what I did that night. I waited for the warmth to come. It came, but it came with a startle. Every time I was about to drift off, I would suddenly and involuntarily jerk awake. Heart racing, sweat beading, I grew more and more fearful of my own body. I guess I wouldn't be winning the game of who can give more in our relationship tonight. I nudged Paul and asked him to give me a priesthood blessing.

I'd had some miraculous experiences with priesthood blessings in my life. I expected no less that night. Paul placed his hands on my head and spoke the words that he felt prompted to say. I remember being told I would be blessed with sleep or rest or something, except, I didn't sleep, not much anyway. It was hard to tell how much I was asleep between stupor and startled jerks. What was going on? Why would I be blessed with sleep and then not sleep? I asked for another blessing the next night, with the same result. Night after night, my fear grew as my body relentlessly rebelled against me. Had I done something wrong? Was Paul not in tune with the spirit when he administered those blessings? Maybe it was because I wasn't studying my scriptures like I should. But how could I? I was a sleep-deprived mother of a toddler and a newborn. Between caring for them, keeping

---

2   A program providing education about the physical processes involved in pregnancy and childbirth as well as methods of managing pain and anxiety throughout.

the house clean, doing laundry, cooking, losing the baby weight, and everything else I had to do, when was I supposed to have the energy to read?

I was scared. I had reached my limit. I could no longer carry the weight of the world on my increasingly fragile shoulders.

In my mind, I kept saying the same prayer over and over.

"Please, Father, please, I just need you to help me sleep, and then I can take care of the rest."

I pleaded with him again and again.

God didn't answer.

So I went to the doctor.

CHAPTER 4

Beguiled

When adversity comes, don't let something you don't fully under-
stand unravel everything you do know.

ELDER KEVIN W. PEARSON

I didn't want to take drugs. Of course, I had learned of many natural remedies over the past three years that could help with sleep, but I was concerned about taking supplements all labeled with the warning "Consult your doctor if you are pregnant or breastfeeding" or "Warning: Not intended for women who are pregnant or lactating." I knew this was just a precaution, as studies for most of these products during pregnancy had never been done. I figured it was safer though to take something that had been studied and FDA approved. After encouraging me to look into sleep therapy, my family doctor assured me that the literature showed Ambien was not likely to get into the breast milk. I didn't have the time or money for specialists and therapy sessions. I figured I would take the sleep aid for a few short weeks, just long enough to get my sleep cycle regulated, and then I would get off.

This was a hard decision for me. It flew in the face of everything I had been learning. But I was desperate for sleep.

I stayed on Ambien for less than one week. Despite what the

literature says, it became obvious to me after the first few days on the sleeping pills that my nursing baby was being affected by them. My once vibrant daughter had become disengaged and sleepy all the time. That wasn't like her, and I knew it was because of the medication. I didn't want to risk any harm to my baby, especially after everything she had been through with meningitis. After five or six days of glorious sleep, I cold turkeyed Ambien for the second time.

Several weeks later, I was even worse than when I first went in. Looking back, it's obvious that before Ambien, I went into the doctor with only one complaint, insomnia. After the Ambien, I developed a laundry list of symptoms, a syndrome created by the very medication that was supposed to help me. Ironically, it had never occurred to either of us to view the Ambien as the culprit for my worsening insomnia and new symptoms. After all, I had only been on it for less than one week and well off of it for several weeks before I made an appointment to discuss my worsening condition.

"Are you feeling depressed? Maybe this is postpartum depression."

I winced as the words I had been trying to avoid for months finally materialized in front of me. I had tried so hard to craft my conversations with Dr. Scott so as to avoid the subject of anxiety and depression. He and I had known each other for ten years. I liked him; he was an osteopath and not your stereotypical self-important doctor with an awkward bedside manner. His slight frame and balding head of black hair lent to his natural air of sensitivity and sincere kindness. I specifically sought out an osteopath when Paul and I moved back to Utah. I wanted a doctor who was open to new thinking, a doctor who would actually listen to me. Dr. Scott was great. He had always been open to any outside-the-box ideas I had when it came to my healthcare. He even offered to visit our home on his way to work the morning after I delivered Lucy. I felt our relationship was one of mutual respect.

"Well, yes I'm depressed, I haven't slept in over a month! I can't read a book, watch TV, or keep food in my stomach. Wouldn't you be depressed? I don't want to medicate normal."

I chalked everything up to not sleeping. I figured the stress of nursing a new baby combined with insomnia was just taking its toll on me. But some symptoms were concerning because they didn't make any sense. Why couldn't I even read a few sentences without it making me dizzy, and sending me running to the bathroom? What about insomnia leads to pelvic pain so severe that I couldn't even walk around the block? Most days, I would lie on the floor for hours, feeling like I was going to blackout every time I stood up. Women I leaned on for respite when Nathaniel was a frantic newborn now brought over food for my family because I couldn't even cook a meal. They offered to take my son to their homes to play with their kids and grandkids while I did my best to care for Lucy. Paul would come home from work to find me on the floor with the baby, dishes in the sink, dirty laundry piled up, and his wife battling with thoughts of suicide. It was something I had never felt before, not even when Ethan died. During that time, Nathaniel also became anxious and started having difficulty sleeping. Our little family was falling apart, and there didn't seem to be any end in sight.

When Dr. Scott brought up the possibility of postpartum depression at that appointment, I knew where he was going with things. The next suggestion would be antidepressants. The little reading I had done on psychiatric medications over the years led me to believe they ultimately resulted in a worsening of the original problem. Pooling serotonin leads to less serotonin. It's just how our bodies adapt to extreme chemical imbalances. I was already dealing with a myriad of inexplicable symptoms. I had no desire to complicate things further. I would wait it out until it got better.

But it didn't get better.

Four months passed.

Meanwhile, Paul drove me to the ophthalmologist to test my eyes, to the hospital to get a CT of my pelvis, an MRI of my brain, an EKG for my heart. I was actually hoping that I had a brain tumor which might explain everything, and validate my complaints. When the tilt table test came back abnormal (the only test that did), the annoyed cardiologist took one look at my wilted demeanor and told me I probably just needed to eat more salt. His response typified the condescension and suspicion I would continue to face from every medical provider I encountered over the next several years. I couldn't really blame them at first. When every test comes back negative, you start to look like a hypochondriac. When you're a woman, worse, a woman who's had a few babies, every emotion, physical ailment, or word that comes out of your mouth is attributed to some sort of emotional imbalance. Why shouldn't it be post-partum depression? There was no test to confirm or deny it. There was only my intuition versus the doctors'.

Everything inside me told me not to take the medications I was being offered for depression and anxiety. I didn't have any concrete reasons as to why. And like my experience as a mother of a son who, at the time, had an undiagnosed illness, I had to defend my choices even to those closest to me. I didn't have the opinion of some medical professional backing up my claims that my son's behavior, sleep, and body were negatively affected for days after a trip to the local fast food restaurant. All I had was the evidence of my experience and the certainty that I had stumbled upon many truths in my search for answers. Likewise, there was something wrong with me, and I knew it wasn't this thing they called depression. It was hard to think clearly so I couldn't give them a good answer; I just knew that the doctors' advice felt wrong. After months of dismissal and proffered psychiatric labels, I began to lose confidence in myself, and in God. Maybe they were right. Maybe I was broken. Maybe God intended to lead me down this path through his silence.

I have beaten myself up many times over the years for giving in and taking the medications I felt were so wrong in so many ways. If I had only waited it out, my injured brain and body would have eventually healed, and life would be so very different now. If only I'd had faith in the blessing Paul gave me that first night of insomnia, the faith to wait and be patient, I would have found sleep eventually. But I didn't know then what I know now. I had no idea that taking Ambien during the three months I was in the hospital on bed rest with Nathaniel meant I would be more susceptible to injury the next time I took it. It's called kindling,[1] and most doctors don't even understand this. I had no idea how lucky I was to have cold turkeyed before with relatively little difficulty. How could I have possibly known that taking Ambien years later, for less than a week, would cause an injury so severe it takes months or even years to heal? How could I know when the prescribing literature says absolutely nothing about this?

---

1   A neuropharmacologic phenomenon that involves sensitization of the nervous system related to repeated exposure to a substance, such as alcohol or benzodiazepines. Clinically, this may present as increased severity of withdrawals on successive use and then discontinuation of those agents. Benzoreform.org

I didn't know then what I know now. I always felt it was my pride and fear that led to my suffering, and I suppose that's partly true in that it led to some poor decisions. But what I did, in taking medication, wasn't a sin. It was a mistake. I transgressed the laws of chemistry or biology or what have you. I've learned to forgive myself for my transgression. Years of being powerless in pretty much every single aspect of my life have taught me the awesome power of acceptance. I've finally learned I will never be superhuman enough to deal with all the bad in the world, but I can lean on superhuman shoulders. Eight years after my last dose of Ambien, I now realize this was the only way I not only had the strength to endure what I did, but also to heal, and use my healing to help others. It's probably the most overlooked miracle that happens all around us every day; when something good is created out of something bad, when weakness is turned into strength.

I wasn't so kind to myself back then. I measured my value as a human being on how clean my home was and how engaged my children were in activities. I knew I was good because I was the person who sought out ways to help others in need. I would take care of their kids or bring them meals. But now I was the person who'd spent four months lying on the floor during the day doing nothing, then pacing around the house all night like a madwoman. My dad started coming down from Sandy whenever he could to drive Nathaniel to and from preschool. My neighbors' charity was wearing thin. Finally, one day, my Relief Society compassionate service leader[2] came to my door and told me she couldn't keep asking people to volunteer to help me

2   Compassionate Service leader is one of the assigned callings women receive as members of the church's Relief Society. Their job is to organize service on behalf of those who are struggling in the ward.

with meals and childcare. I told her I understood and thanked her for everything she and others had done for my family and me. Paul's friend told him how he had experienced a breakdown at one point that seemed very similar to what I was going through. He said he was given two medications to get him through that crisis. One he was told to taper off after a few weeks, which he did no problem. The other he got off of after several months. He encouraged us to give the doctor a try. I couldn't take it anymore. I was so miserable; I was willing to do anything to get some relief.

The next day I called the doctor's office. Dr. Scott was out of town, so I saw his colleague. He gave me a couple sheets of paper with questions for me to answer. They asked me things like, on a scale of 1-to-10 have you had thoughts of harming others, suicidal thoughts, how often do you cry, worry about the future, etc. I put a zero on thoughts of suicide. Yes, it had crossed my mind some nights as I paced in between my bathroom and bedroom that my family might be better off without me, but it wasn't something I wanted to act on. It was more of this terrifying voice in my ear telling me over and over it was an option. It scared me. One night, I admitted to Paul what was going on inside my head. As the words came out of my mouth, I felt ashamed. He didn't know what to say. How could he? I sounded like some attention-seeking drama queen. But what else could I do? If I didn't talk about these thoughts, they would continue to fester inside of me, eating away until I was too weak to resist.

I didn't want to be labeled suicidal though, not on some worksheet that might follow me throughout the rest of my life on my medical records. I figured anyone trapped for months in a body that was going crazy with no sleep would probably feel the same. I didn't deserve to be judged for that. I answered the rest of the test as best I could, considering I could barely read and interpret the words on the page. It hurt my brain to think that hard. Where was the question for that symptom? Oh, difficulty concentrating. Yeah, except this went way beyond that. This was like someone taking a hand mixer to my brain every 10 seconds. My neurons were constantly forced to take detours to get to the end of a thought.

The doctor tallied up the points as if I had just taken a pop quiz on the American Revolution.

"These scores are pretty high. You definitely have major depressive disorder and an anxiety disorder. Since you're so low energy, I think it would be a good idea to take an SNRI[3] instead of an SSRI. Antidepressants can take a few weeks to start working though, so I'm going to prescribe you another medication to help until that kicks in. It's only meant for short term use."

Right, that made sense. Our friend had said the same thing.

"How long will I stay on the antidepressant?"

"Some people get off after six months, maybe up to a year."

"Ok, because I don't want to be on this forever."

"That's fine. Just make sure to taper[4] off the short-term medication first."

I was given one milligram of Lorazepam (Ativan) along with an antidepressant called Effexor. That week I went to my parents' house, so they could help me with the kids while Paul was out of town. I lay

---

3   Serotonin-norepinephrine reuptake inhibitor are similar to SSRI's (selective serotonin reuptake inhibitors) which are the most commonly prescribed antidepressants.

4   A gradual reduction off a dose of medication.

down on my mom's couch to rest. Forty-five minutes later, I woke up from a nap. I couldn't believe it! I had actually slept, and in the middle of the day no less! "The antidepressant must have already been kicking in!" I thought.

I improved slightly over the next few weeks. But I was still not a fully functional human being. After one month, I followed up with Dr. Scott. I was asked another series of questions as he probed various points on my body from head to toe. All of them were painful. I was sleeping a few hours a night now, but not enough. I still had all the same symptoms, just less severe. He diagnosed me with fibromyalgia and switched me from Effexor to Cymbalta.

"What about the Lorazepam? Don't I need to start tapering off of that soon?"

"You're doing better with it. Let's leave well enough alone."

"But I'm still not sleeping much. I'm still pretty miserable, actually."

"Let's add another milligram of Lorazepam and see how you feel on that."

He changed my dose to 2 mg Lorazepam every night.

All of a sudden, I felt better! I got a full seven hours of unbroken sleep for the first time in five months. Not only that, but now I was magically able to clean the house, take the kids to the park, go to church, read books, and watch movies. I felt like me again. It was like I'd been resurrected from the dead. I figured the antidepressant was finally doing its job. I figured I really had suffered some kind of mental breakdown. I had endured abuse, poverty, and the loss of a child. But after all those weeks worrying about Paul and Lucy and Nathaniel all while trying to nurse and recover from giving birth, I had finally fallen apart. Apparently, I wasn't as strong as I thought I was. I obviously needed the medication to get through this crisis. I would taper off the Lorazepam after I had a chance to recover from all those months of being unwell, and then get off the Cymbalta after that.

Acceptance of my need for these medications and that they could do some good felt like a betrayal of my entire life's philosophy. I didn't know what to believe anymore. Everything I thought I knew about health and healing had just flown out the window, a window that would suddenly shut without warning and remain that way for five years.

CHAPTER 5

Dreamless

"Oh the nerves, the nerves; the mysteries of this machine called man! Oh, the little that unhinges it, poor creatures that we are!"

CHARLES DICKENS, THE CHIMES

If I could use one word to describe the next three and a half years, what comes to mind is "dreamless." Literally, you don't dream on benzos.[1] While they knock you out, tranquilizers don't give you "true" sleep because they prevent you from getting into a deep REM cycle. I don't remember having had a single dream while taking Lorazepam, but it did have its benefits. I could go and go all day, take my little white pill right before bed, wait for that floaty feeling to kick in, then go right to sleep. I couldn't sleep in anymore though and, in fact, I never got a full eight hours sleep. But during that time I never had to worry about having a sleepless night. Every night was a guaranteed seven hours of blissful unconsciousness, no matter what.

There were other dreams that vanished too, just as our situation began to improve. Paul was able to build us a new home on a piece of property we had purchased with credit. We didn't have much, but

---

1   Benzodiazepines: A class of tranquilizers most commonly used to treat anxiety that includes Xanax, Ativan, Valium, and Klonopin among others.

we did have great credit, and that got us through the recession. Paul would take out loans to buy repossessed cars (there were many back then) and fix them up. We were able to sell all the cars we purchased and were never late on a payment. Once the economy picked up, we were able to get even bigger loans for things like land and materials which we would use to build homes. We set up our own construction business. We had residual income from the renter at our old house now, and it looked like we were on our way to living the American Dream. We could actually buy things we wanted and perhaps even go on a family vacation.

But after moving into our new house in 2011, a year after I started taking medication, we did very little. Despite our newly acquired financial freedom, I never made plans to go anywhere or do anything fun as a family. It wasn't a conscious decision on my part. It was just that planning anything beyond my daily routine was outside of my vision. I preferred to stay home, doing little activities with my kids and the neighbor's kids.

There were only three homes on our corner of the neighborhood, and I had become something of a block mom. I would organize playtime games and activities for all the kids, usually outside or in our unfinished basement. It was a good thing we weren't dependent on charity anymore to fill our pantry because two or three tweens could empty my cupboards in one visit! We bought Nathaniel and Lucy a trampoline that Christmas. It ended up being more of a neighborhood trampoline, and that was fine with me. I had a purpose. I enjoyed being able to help other people again, like the single working mom on the corner or our next door neighbor who was overwhelmed with her third pregnancy.

Life was good, even if I never felt like playing the hand-me-down piano Paul had purchased for my birthday that year. Occasionally I would force myself to pull out some sheet music and sit on the bench and play, but it was as if all the music inside me had gone silent. I was just going through the motions. I didn't feel like singing either. Even though I had been offered a solo in the local tabernacle Christmas production, my inability to control the face twitching and voice cracking I'd struggled with over the years overwhelmed any desire I now had to perform.

I found other hobbies to fill my time. Mostly I did crafts that I read about online. I learned to sew, quilt, and repurpose hand-me-downs from the local thrift store. I would stay up late into the night sewing Halloween costumes or a blouse. Then I would take my little white pill and pass out before Paul could approach me for physical affection.

Once, I had been the ideal Christian woman, full of do good energy who cheerfully accepted every church assignment given to her. Now, I found it difficult to handle lessons for the Activity Day girls[2] at church who were assigned to come to my home each week. I liked teaching them, but having two little ones running around the house or clinging to me for attention while trying to teach a lesson was too unpredictable, uncontrollable, imperfect and that bothered me in a way it never would have before. The woman who used to go out for karaoke nights with girlfriends or impulsively drive up the mountain to hike with her baby boy strapped to her back, dog on a leash, had been replaced with a crafty homebody, who binged on a dozen

---

2   Girls 8-11 in the church who get together once every other week with two adults assigned to be their leaders for lessons and activities. Similar to Cub Scouts.

or two homemade sugar cookies every night. Running four miles or the intense weight lifting I used to do almost always led to a massive headache so, naturally, my exercise habits changed too. Then I developed my first case of what eventually became chronic bacterial vaginosis, something I later found was directly related to the Lorazepam. My emotions and my body were not the same. What happened to the powerful, passionate woman who could turn dreams into reality?

Like Joseph of Egypt, I was a dreamer of dreams. In waking moments or in sleep, an image would form in my mind, and that image would become a reality. When I was younger, I would quite literally have a dream about the person I was dating. I would see what our lives would be like together and, well, until Paul came along, this always ended in my inexplicably and suddenly breaking up with a somewhat bewildered young man.

I had a dream when I was 16. Well, it was part dream, part nightmare. The summer before my junior year in high school, I pondered on the two Young Women[3] personal projects I needed to complete before the end of my senior year. These were like senior or Eagle Scout projects where you commit to spending 100 hours working on a goal. The project was to be based on one or more of the seven Young Women values which are faith, divine nature, individual worth, knowledge, choice and accountability, good works, and integrity. As I thought about the options available to me, I realized that much of my divine nature was apparent in the talents I had worked to develop over the

---

3   The Young Women, an organization of The Church of Jesus Christ of Latter-day Saints, provides instruction, encouragement, growth opportunities, development, and support in living the gospel of Jesus Christ for female Church members ages 12 through 17.

years. I saw myself performing a piano/vocal recital on stage for a large audience. The idea was terrifying because by the middle of my sophomore year, I had begun to develop a kind of stutter when I was singing. My eyes would involuntarily close, my face would distort, and my voice would suddenly crack or make this weird glottal sound. I was rarely able to get through an entire song without having at least one or two of these spasms. The last thing I wanted to do was stand on a stage in front of hundreds of people watching me have these "twitches" as I called them. But the image in my mind wouldn't go away.

The next spring, I stood on the stage of the concert hall at the local college. Dressed in black, I flawlessly worked my way through ten piano pieces. From Chopin to Mozart and finally Bumble Boogie, all were performed from memory. After the intermission, I came out in white, this time to sing classical songs in Italian and German alongside a few Broadway pieces and one Irish ballad. I couldn't have been more nervous. My performance was anything but flawless. I cracked, I twitched and blinked, and that weird sound my throat made when all that happened, was amplified by a microphone and impeccable acoustics. But I did it anyway, and I was praised for the beauty of my voice, even with all its flaws. I never liked watching the second half of my recital on video. I would watch the piano part and then turn it off before I came out on stage to sing. Other people may have enjoyed the vocal recital, but I didn't. I knew I could do better.

The stutter continued to interfere with my ability to perform, but I was still cast in community productions of *Pirates of Penzance* and *Joseph and the Amazing Technicolor Dream Coat*. When I went to BYU, I decided to focus on dance instead of voice. I'd had years of ballet, tap and jazz instruction and decided to try out for Living Legends. I spent the summer of '97 learning a Jalisco dance routine. Even though I'm Hispanic and grew up in a very old town rich with Latin culture and parents who speak Spanish, I had never really embraced my heritage before. In fact, I often felt a sense of shame over it. "We're not dirty Mexicans," my Grandma would say. The one whose name was changed from Eurcinia to Lucy when she went to school because the teacher couldn't pronounce her name. This was the first time I had ever felt proud of my ethnicity! To dance with Living Legends, you have to prove you are at least one quarter Latin American, Native American, or Polynesian before you can even audition. Due to my ethnicity and my audition, I made the final cut. I spent the next two years performing all across the U.S. during the school year then, in the summer, we would travel abroad and perform throughout the world.

I loved performing. It was my passion. I could go and go without a break. It didn't matter if it was after three hours of practice, or four hours on the bus followed by a mini-performance at a high school and a night show afterward. My soul fed off the energy of the music, and there was always enough to spare. After performances and assemblies, we would go out into the audience to visit with people or into the classrooms to speak with the students. I saw lives changed and hearts opened by the simple act of sharing my culture and faith with the people who came to watch. I learned to love and accept myself and others so much more through that experience.

This translated into my career as an educator. After moving from North Carolina to Utah, I spent two years teaching elementary PE at a Title I school. In the middle of my first year, I had an inspired idea of putting together a dance festival for the students and parents. I'd had a vision. Each grade would perform a dance from one of the cultures represented at our school. I had no idea how this was going to happen as many of the kids were transient, and many more of the parents didn't speak English. But all the teachers were so thrilled not to have to spend their precious class time putting together their usual yearly hoedown, that everyone contributed materials. They even made their students available for extra practices during the school day. The music and computer specialty teachers worked with me in teaching the kids songs from and researching the culture they were representing. Kindergarten did an Asian ribbon dance, first grade performed La Raspa from Mexico, and second grade learned a Native American round dance. Third grade learned a hula, fourth the maypole, fifth a dance from Ghana, Africa, and sixth was Maori. I saw friendships form, and barriers dissolve. Children who had once separated themselves by language, culture, and skin color now embraced each other out of a newfound fascination for the cultures in which they had been immersed. The feeling the day of the festival was amazing. The teachers all wanted to make it a yearly tradition. Unfortunately, the next year I had to resign before the end of the school year when I was put on bed rest with Nathaniel.

After quitting my job to become a full-time mom, I continued to find ways to make music and dance part of my life. There were always opportunities to perform with local artists and in the church. When I didn't have a public venue, I would find an unoccupied church piano or a friend with one. Then I'd cart over a stack about a foot tall of sheet music and sit and play and sing for hours. I started teaching Nathaniel piano. Music was my comfort, my soul, and when I wasn't focused on it, I was always able to find something else to be passionate about. In this case, I added nutrition to my list of interests. My husband and I started working out together. I read every book I could about nutrition, and even a couple Paul recommended on finance and business. In 2008 I wrote and self-published a recipe book. I opened up a small health business with a friend. My dreams were expanding. For the first time in my life, I truly believed I was capable of accomplishing anything I put my mind to. I wanted to become a midwife, an herbalist, a speaker, a coach, a nutritionist, a chiropractor ... anything I dreamed was possible!

But starting in 2010, dreams ceased to be a part of my life, disappearing as suddenly from my consciousness as they had from my unconscious sleep. I was a different person, and that person just didn't care anymore.

CHAPTER 6
Heartless

*"...Never shall I forget those moments which murdered my God
and my soul and turned my dreams to dust. Never shall I forget
these things, even if I am condemned to live as long as God Himself.
Never."*

ELIE WIESEL, NIGHT

Paul and I began to fight more and more despite counseling. He tried
so hard to find ways to repair our sexual relationship, which had already been injured by the darts and arrows of weaknesses we each
brought into our marriage. But years of heartache related not only to
intimacy but also to physical complications from my first pregnancy
and now the effects of the medications, made it so that even thinking
about sex with my husband left me both numb and angry. No matter
how illogical or unfair it may have been, I felt that any efforts on his
part to help me out were merely a reflection of his own selfish desires
and had very little to do with my needs. It's like I couldn't feel anything towards my husband other than tolerance at best. Paul was the
only man I had ever given myself to. Not that I was prudish in any way
when we got married. I was simply raised a Latter-day Saint, and I had
been taught and had the desire to wait until marriage to have sex.

Of course, I had been attracted to many men both before and after my marriage. But I never allowed myself to dwell for too long on any thoughts or to be in any situations that might lead me to compromise my standards. There was a clear line, and I promised myself never to cross it. However, that line started to blur and became increasingly blurry during the next couple of years. I found myself daydreaming about encounters with men of my acquaintance. These weren't men that I particularly liked or would even have normally found attractive. They were simply present. I found it difficult not to think about calling or texting them. I was excited, motivated even, by the thought of being desirable to someone else, of being sexually in control of someone in make-believe because I couldn't control the people around me in real life.

I cringe to think of how many times I could have ruined my marriage. I don't know if I can blame it one hundred percent on the drugs. But there was definitely an element of lowered inhibition and obsessive thinking that slowly unraveled the chord that connected me to my husband, and to myself. I didn't realize obsessiveness and lack of inhibition along with hypersexuality are common side effects of antidepressants and benzodiazepines. I wasn't even aware of these changes in my personality. I was blind to the numbness that had taken over, dulled my compassion, and replaced understanding with perfectionism. Sadly, my chemically altered personality led to more heartache than a strained relationship with my husband.

After Ethan died, Paul used to take me to pet stores both to get me out of the house and so I could have something small and warm to hold in my arms. One night, we happened upon a lady with a litter of Maltese and Shih Tzu puppies. While the other puppies distractedly sniffed around and played with each other, a little runt Maltese came up to me and immediately cuddled up. I had a hard time leaving him when it was time to go. When Paul inquired about the litter, he found they had been born on December 18th, Ethan's birthday. It was inevitable. We had to get the dog. The owner, whose daughter had delivered a stillborn baby a few years back, sympathized with us and offered to sell us the puppy for a price far below what she was asking. Paul and I left the pet shop that evening with a little white ball of fluff so tiny he fit in my front pocket, but who was so gassy he could clear a room. We started calling him Maxiumus Flatulus, a joke meant to be both literal and ironic.

On our way home, the three of us stopped by Wal-Mart and picked up a few puppy necessities along with a book on how to train your Maltese. Max became my unofficial therapy dog. A creature so impossibly small, when I would walk him down the street, people would stop and say, "where are the batteries?" Yet Max filled my whole world. He gave me the courage to face the sorrowful looks and awkward condolences of the friends I encountered. I trained him to ring a bell to go outside, poop and pee on command, roll over, drop things when I said "poison" and even put his toys in a basket. He was the best trained little puppy in town. I loved Max. That's why it's so heartbreaking to remember how unable I was to care about him in the years following my diagnoses.

After moving into our new house, Paul and I began to notice that Max was hiding a lot under the couch and vomiting. We took him in to the vet who, after a few tests told us there was nothing they could do for him. By this point, Max was walking all wobbly and couldn't seem to go in a straight line. It was sad to see, especially since he was only six years old, relatively young for a small dog. But I didn't feel the need to do anything more to preserve my dog's life. We had taken him to the vet, and if it was his time to go, well, it's not like the kids were all that attached to him. Max had always been my dog, not theirs. Besides, the idea of dealing with another death in the family was just too much to think about. Paul thought about it for me. He went back to the vet several times and then finally insisted they give Max an IV and a strong course of antibiotics, just in case. Max's symptoms reminded Paul of Lucy and her meningitis. If there was something attacking Max's brain, then he had to at least try. After three days of treatment, Max unexpectedly and remarkably recovered. They started calling him Miracle Max at the vet's, and we were happy to have him home.

The next time though, it was cancer. The antibiotics gave us an extra year with Max. Then, at the beginning of 2014, several months after we moved into our second home Paul built, a large tumor developed on Max's leg. We decided to get it removed, but the vet let us know that it was impossible to remove every cancerous cell and that it would almost certainly return to claim Max's life. Max passed later that December during my first year of withdrawing from Cymbalta and Lorazepam. I was in the deepest, darkest place in my life, and incapable of even thinking of anything other than my own suffering. Not until the pharmaceutical shroud was lifted and my eyes adjusted to the light would the true loss of my beloved Max hit me full force in the face. It didn't even occur to me when he died that he and Ethan had both passed away at Christmas time. In 2015, two years after Max's passing, I finally felt his loss. Without the drugs to obscure the pain of my memories, I felt as though I had lost Ethan all over again. It felt like I had lost both Ethan and Max that month. The grief was indescribable and the guilt even more so. How could I have cared so little about the passing of a soul who saved me from despair with his love? What kind of a monster had I become?

I grieved another loss that Christmas, the loss of the woman I used to be.

CHAPTER 7

Jumping Off

Let me tell you somethin' you already know. The world ain't all sunshine and rainbows. It is a very mean and nasty place and it will beat you to your knees and keep you there permanently if you let it. You, me, or nobody is gonna hit as hard as life. But it ain't how hard you hit; it's about how hard you can get hit, and keep moving forward. How much you can take, and keep moving forward. That's how winning is done!

ROCKY BALBOA (2006 FILM)

"Aren't you exhausted?"

My mother-in-law asked. She was visiting from Las Vegas in the summer of 2012. Delores was helping me watch the kids while I packed. We had contracted out our second home to renters, but our new home build was behind schedule, and it would be a few months before we could move into our new house. The plan was to put most of our belongings in storage and rent somewhere until it was finished. I should have been exhausted. I had two energetic little children, I had been packing the entire house by myself all week, and this was the second move for us in two years. I suddenly realized that it was kind of unnatural for me not to be feeling somewhat overwhelmed or tired.

That thought picked away at my brain over the next week as we finished moving. I figured I was probably numbed by the time release SNRI continuously flowing through my system. I knew that the Cymbalta hadn't been doing me much good. I was ten pounds heavier than normal, chronically constipated, and still in constant pain. I did a bit of research and asked my doctor about using progesterone as a treatment for many of the side effects I had developed, including lack of libido. We decided to use a natural form of the hormone that I would get compounded at the pharmacy. My mood and pain seemed to improve a bit after starting the progesterone, but it was hard to tell if it was making much of a difference. I didn't believe the diagnosis of major depressive disorder I had been given was ever legitimate. After all, I got better almost as soon as I started sleeping. That had more to do with the Lorazepam than the Cymbalta. Besides, I never liked the idea of being on an SNRI drug. I had wanted to get off it as soon as possible, but my doctor told me I needed to get off the Lorazepam before tapering the antidepressant.

Many times, I would try to cut off one quarter of the teeny white sleeping pill as Dr. Scott had instructed. I would suffer through the restless sleep and insomnia for a few nights until it became too much, then give up and take a whole pill one night. I thought most of my difficulty during these attempts was due to the lack of sleep. I didn't understand how much I was also crippled by unnatural chemical fear when cutting my dose. It didn't feel like fear, and I didn't understand or know how to recognize anxiety back then. I thought I was just sleep-deprived. Only the perspective of hindsight has allowed me to recognize the symptoms of withdrawal that manifested as irrational fear, anxiety, and an inability to perceive things as they truly are. But the symptoms I experienced after each attempt to reduce my dose were severe enough that I began to doubt I would ever be able to get off of Lorazepam.

After giving some thought to my health, my marriage, and my mother-in-law's question, I decided it was better to get off the Cymbalta now, even if I was still on a benzodiazepine. Dr. Scott told me to open the capsule and count out the little beads. The plan was to reduce the dose by a small amount every other day, then reduce by that amount every day the next week, following this pattern until I was off. He told me to take it slow, at least a few months. I implemented this new regimen as we settled into our temporary new home. The taper went better than expected! I hardly noticed the reductions; in fact, I was feeling great, almost euphoric. I began to take the kids and the dog for long walks in the double stroller I delighted in the little two-bedroom farmhouse with its tiny kitchen and great big yard. Sitting under the shade of the front porch during Lucy's nap time each day, I relished the quiet as Nathaniel played at my feet with his Legos. Later in the afternoon the kids and I would pick raspberries and currants from the bushes and apples from trees. That was a good summer.

In a few months, it was time to move to the next town over and into our new house. Somewhere along the way, I suddenly stopped the progesterone. I can't exactly say why I did this. I may have thought that it wasn't really having the effect I hoped it would. Also, there were so many other things to focus on with registering Nathaniel for kindergarten and fixing up our new home and yard. Maybe I just lost it in the move. Either way, it took years before I made the connection between my sudden decline after the move and my progesterone cold turkey. The fibromyalgia pain got worse and worse, and the bathroom scale crept higher and higher. I felt depressed and exhausted for no reason. After dinner, I would often go upstairs to rest from the pain and fatigue, only to find myself waking up an hour or two later, face down, feet dangling off the edge of the bed. I guessed I was wrong about not needing the Cymbalta after all. I was a mess!

I had gotten so close to getting off, down to just 15 mg. But I promptly went back up to 60 mg. That's when my health really deteriorated. I was still depressed, still in pain, and now I was even more exhausted. Worst of all, I started packing on the weight, and my blood pressure was getting dangerously high, problems I'd never even remotely experienced before taking psychiatric medications. No matter how much I exercised or reduced calories, I just kept getting bigger and bigger. After a few months, I was hovering around second to third trimester pregnancy weight. I was incredibly frustrated. What was the point of taking this medication if it didn't help with any of the things it was supposed to treat? And I was getting fat! I didn't even want to bother with a long drawn out taper this time. I was just going to jump off my medication.

And jump I did, right into crazy.

I felt crazy. Crazy and miserable. My mind was in a frenzy. I was crying, shaking, pacing. I was frightened by this terrifying sensation I would get, where it felt like someone suddenly jerked my head back and shut off my brain for a split second. It was as if I had a millisecond of a seizure. It was eerily disorienting. Paul looked up Cymbalta withdrawal online and found that others described this symptom as "head zaps." "That's exactly it!" I cried. "It's like someone is sending a jolt of electricity through your brain for an instant." I was afraid to turn my head or suddenly focus my eyes in a different direction because this would usually trigger a head zap. I wanted to scream. The shakes were uncontrollable. I imagine I looked much like someone going through alcohol detox.

At least some of the weight was coming off, and I was still sleeping at night. I had the Lorazepam to thank for the latter. Even with the seven hours of nightly respite, I continued having a difficult time for the first month. Then it turned into two. I was supposed to be volunteering once a week as a room mom in my son's kindergarten class, but I could hardly make it out of bed in the mornings. "Mrs. Pedersen, we really need your help on Fridays. If you have to miss a day, can you please let us know ahead of time so we can find a substitute?" I couldn't let them know. I didn't know myself how bad I was going to be from one day to the next or how long this would last. I had difficulty with both my body and my brain. Logical decisions like: "call your kid's teacher to let them know you won't be showing up," simply flew over my head.

One morning, knowing Lucy needed to get out of the house, I decided I should set up a playdate for my daughter, despite the struggle I knew I would have in accomplishing such a simple task. We drove, rather than walked around the corner to a friend's house. I sat there in the basement, trying to feign normal conversation. The mom was a spunky, attractive redheaded mother of four. We knew each other from church, but we'd never had any deep conversations before then. Audrey could tell I wasn't feeling well and, after she asked me what was going on, I opened up to her about my antidepressant cold turkey. I told her how difficult I was finding it to function. I even told her about feeling kind of crazy. "That sounds like anxiety," she said. "Really?" I was surprised to hear that term applied to my list of symptoms. I had always thought anxiety was phobias and being too afraid to speak in public. "I had no idea anxiety could be physical!" The words sounded stupid as they left my mouth. Of course anxiety was physical. I had just never given it that much thought.

Audrey confided in me that she'd had quite severe anxiety after one of her pregnancies. She developed terrible insomnia as a result. Then she told me about a program she found that helped her work through this period in her life. It was an anxiety and depression program she ordered online. She took me upstairs and pulled down a box from her closet filled with several workbooks and some CDs. She told me it had saved her life and helped her start sleeping again. "This is like the gospel for anxiety," Audrey exclaimed. "It's so wonderful; I really think everyone should learn the stuff they teach in this program." That sounded great to me. I wanted to start right then. I asked her if I could borrow the first CD. She gave me the first two.

I listened to the introduction the next day. The day after that was Sunday, and I felt too weak to go to church with my family. I asked Paul if he could take the kids by himself. It was a beautiful, sunny fall day. I sat down on the lawn in our backyard, wrapped in a blanket, with a piece of paper and a pen. Sans manual, I followed the suggestions on the CD and wrote down all the thoughts that were causing me to feel dizzy or shaky as they rapidly fired across my brain. Then, I worked my way backward from those thoughts until I found the underlying fears that were the source of my body's response. Once I did that, I was able to write down the "truth" or the words that I needed to tell myself to replace those fears.

I was amazed at how productive that hour of writing was for me. I uncovered so many debilitating fears, and negative thoughts that I never even realized were a part of my subconscious. I was never one to talk about feelings. I always found labels like anxiety and depression demeaning. But now I jumped feet first into a whole new way of looking at myself and the people around me, and it was liberating. My *Attacking Anxiety and Depression* program by Lucinda Bassett eventually arrived in the mail. Daily, over the next few weeks, my "crazy" improved astronomically. It's like I could feel my brain rewiring as I learned to replace the false narratives with true ones. I found deeply held beliefs that I realized had been holding me back in many ways even before the Cymbalta fried my brain. But the majority of them really were a product of the three years I had spent on mind-altering medications. How I wished I'd had this resource before I ever went into the doctor with insomnia! I would have never taken the Ambien.

Even with the *Attacking Anxiety and Depression* course, I still found myself uncontrollably shaky at times. It didn't seem to be connected to any thoughts or fears on my part. One day, I went into the kitchen and grabbed a roll as an afternoon snack. I felt myself almost immediately begin to shake. Oh my gosh! Were the carbohydrates making me do that? I went over to the kitchen cabinet and pulled down one of the weight loss supplements my husband had been using. I had read the ingredients on the label a few months back and remembered that it contained insulin regulating minerals and herbs like chromium and Gymnema sylvestre. I took one pill rather than the recommended two as I was wary about dropping my blood sugar too drastically. Within 20 minutes, the shakiness had subsided, and I felt remarkably stable. It made sense that the Cymbalta made my insulin go as screwy as my brain, that would at least partly explain why I had put on so much weight. I felt so awful eating carbs that I decided it wasn't worth it to eat grains or sugar anymore. I cut them completely out of my diet along with most dairy. The shakiness left and, in a few weeks, about 20 pounds followed it out the door.

Even though I felt somewhat delicate over the next few months, in many ways, I felt better than ever. I was getting stronger day by day, and every week, I would push past my limitations to do and plan things I had not even realized I'd wanted to try before. We took the kids to a snow tube lift in Heber City. I reached out to a friend who was a professional singer and asked her if she could coach the "classical" out of me so I could start performing in more modern venues. I volunteered to play a special piano number in church. I began to feel like anything was possible again, even more so now, because now I understood how to attack anxiety and live without fear.

Next step on the road to healing, freedom from Lorazepam.

CHAPTER 8

Poisoned Fruit

When through the deep waters I call thee to go,
The rivers of sorrow shall not thee o'erflow
For I will be with thee, thy troubles to bless,
And sanctify to thee thy deepest distress.

HYMNS NO. 85 HOW FIRM A FOUNDATION

We knew it would be hard. It was the spring of 2014, and I was finally ready to tackle the Lorazepam. I'd had insomnia for months after my Ambien cold turkey, so Paul and I had an idea of what to expect when I decided to taper off the benzo. From what I had studied, z-drugs like Lunesta and Ambien were so similar to benzodiazepines like Ativan (Lorazepam), Klonopin, Xanax, and Valium that they were basically the same thing. The experience should be similar; only this time, we would be prepared. The plan was to get help with the kids for a few months while I worked my way off the tranquilizer. Paul was at a point with the business where he could be home more to help with the kids anyway. It was good timing, especially since we really wanted to have another baby. I was prepared to convalesce, to give my mind and body the time and space to heal without the guilt of not being supermom every single day. It would just be a few months out of our lives, and then we could go on as planned, with the kids looking forward to a little brother or sister in the near future.

For some reason, in the back of my mind, I thought that being pregnant would be a good motivation for me to finally get off the benzodiazepine. I was finally feeling strong enough after my Cymbalta cold turkey to face withdrawal again, and pregnancy was always such a joyous period in my life. I always felt healthier when pregnant than not. It just seemed like there wasn't much need to be careful since we already wanted to have another child. I would be off the medication soon anyway ...

"You need to get off the Lorazepam right now," Dr. Scott said a few weeks later with a warning tone in his voice. I made an appointment to see him after the pregnancy test came up positive, early of course. As usual, my hormones kicked into high gear from day one of conception.

"Benzodiazepines can cause birth defects within the first 12 weeks,"[1] he cautioned.

"I know," I said with a sinking feeling of guilt, "but I can't cut it by one quarter like before. I want to cut it by one eighth a week and see how that goes." Dr. Scott reluctantly agreed.

I was already feeling pretty miserable. I had just cut an eighth of my pill that week. I was also dealing with a nasty sinus infection that a previous prescription for antibiotics hadn't cured. Actually, I quit taking the antibiotics after only a couple of doses because I thought I'd had an allergic reaction to them. My brain was reeling from the benzo

---

1   Current research shows that while benzodiazepines may not necessarily be teratogenic, they are strongly linked with spontaneous abortion (miscarriage).

reduction, and I couldn't remember the name of the antibiotic when I went back in to follow up with the doctor. So I told him:

"Whatever you prescribe just make sure it's not the one you gave me last time, I think I'm allergic. I swelled up and got a fever. It was super painful."

"Do you remember if it was this one? Or this one?" Dr. Scott asked, pointing to his chart. I couldn't for the life of me make heads or tails of the computer screen. The taper was already kicking my butt. I wasn't even a quarter of the way off my 2 mg pill, and it was already every bit as hard as the Ambien cold turkey I'd experienced three years ago. Plus the pelvic pain was ridiculously intense. Was my pelvis already expanding that much with this pregnancy? I figured pregnancy in my thirties must just be a totally different game.

Dr. Scott asked me again to point out which antibiotic was the problem. Why couldn't he figure this out? He was the doctor! "I don't know, all I know is I don't want to be on anything for too long, especially now that I'm pregnant."

"Ok, I'll prescribe you Ciprofloxacin again. It works fast, and I think you did ok with that one."

One and a half years later, I painfully read through the medical records I had requested from Premier Family Medical. It physically hurt to read them. I had to do it with one eye shut, head cocked to one side, squinting through my other eye. "I was given a fluoroquinolone twice?!" I shouted as I scanned the records from 2014. I had thought the hell of the past year had all been related to the tranquilizers I had been prescribed, the Lorazepam, Ambien, and Valium. Now I suddenly realized I had been floxed twice while pregnant, and on benzos. I eventually learned what being floxed meant through the online benzo withdrawal support community. But I honestly didn't remember the episodes with the Ciprofloxacin until I read through my records. Then I read this in a benzodiazepine withdrawal manual written by one of the world's leading authorities on the subject.

Antibiotics for some reason, sometimes seem to aggravate withdrawal symptoms. However, one class of antibiotics, the quinolones, actually displace benzodiazepines from their binding sites on GABA-receptors. These can precipitate acute withdrawal in people taking or tapering from benzodiazepines. It may be necessary to take antibiotics during benzodiazepine withdrawal but if possible the quinolones should be avoided. (There are at least six different quinolones – ask your doctor if in doubt). The Ashton Manual Supplement 2011:

Of course, I didn't know any of this at the time, and neither did my doctor. The second time I took Cipro, the reaction was even worse. I had a fever, pain, swelling, a rash, and uncontrollable shaking. I was crying frantically as I held onto the side of my bed. I found myself trying to explain my reasons for being so terrified to my husband, but I was unable to reason it out myself. All I knew was that I had a deep in the marrow of my bones kind of pain I'd never had before. I knew something was terribly, terribly wrong and I was worried about the baby, so I simply stopped the Cipro after one dose. It's possible that saved my life. I didn't learn until much later how deadly this kind of reaction could be.

Fluoroquinolones are broad-spectrum antibiotics, including the most widely used of these which are ciprofloxacin, levofloxacin and moxifloxacin. The most serious reactions caused by this class of medication include toxicities of the central nervous system, cardio-vascular system, and the musculoskeletal system.

NCBI

Clin Pract. 2012 Oct 12; 2(4): e87.

Published online 2012 Nov 28. doi: 10.4081/cp.2012.e87

Fluoroquinolone Toxicity Syndrome/Floxing includes damage to connective tissue (tendons, ligaments, cartilage, fascia, etc.) throughout the body, damage to the nervous systems (central, peripheral and autonomic), and more. The damage done by fluoroquinolone antibiotics can destroy a person's quality of life or even kill them. FloxieHope.com

Ravaged by the brutal natures of the fluoroquinolone and benzo-diazepine, I was too sick to make a follow up appointment with Dr. Scott. To this day I have no idea if what I experienced those first few months of withdrawal was due to the Lorazepam, the Cipro, and/or the reaction to having both in my system at the same time. All I know is that by the time I cut another one eighth of a mg from my pill, I suffered from an agony worse than anything I had experienced in getting off Cymbalta or Ambien.

I was mentally and physically disabled to the point where I could no longer drive. I didn't know how I was going to make it all the way up to Salt Lake anymore for the gospel choir practices I had been attending. We had a performance coming up, and I desperately wanted to be able to sing for it. Many of the singers were professional or semiprofessional artists. It was an incredible collection of local talent. Even though I was a novice at singing gospel, I had generously been given a small solo part. For the first time since high school, I was singing without cracking or twitching. Thanks to my vocal coaching, I was finally free to sing exactly like I had always wanted. It was incredibly liberating, being able to sing every range of emotion I felt without restraint. I didn't want to give that up just because of a few months of withdrawal. I offered to let a couple of my younger choir friends drive my car if they would carpool with me to practice.

The drive was torture. At the practice, I found it difficult to talk to people or look anyone in the eye. All I could do was breathe, in and out, in and out, and sing. Amazingly, I had the strength to sing, even though I felt like I might pass out at any minute. Actually, I wished I could pass out. It would be a relief from the disorientation, pain, and suffocating fear. Unfortunately, I couldn't pass out, but I could sing. It was the one part of me that still existed outside my prison of pain. The choir director sat down next to me after the practice. "We got permission to sing one or two songs as a prelude for the singles' ward sacrament meeting this Sunday. Which ones do you think would be most appropriate?" She ran a few titles by me. I was embarrassed to admit that I couldn't remember which song went with which title. What was the melody of that one? What did the words say? I couldn't put it all together into anything that made sense. I did my best to make polite responses and sound coherent. I needed to get out of there. I needed to get home, back to the safety and quiet of my bedroom.

It was two weeks since my first cut, and I was down by a quarter of a pill. According to my doctor, I had already been on the benzodiazepine too long with this baby. I determined I would just have to cut an eighth of a pill every two weeks instead of weekly and the devil take the consequences. I simply didn't have the strength to battle a bigger and badder beast every seven days. That night I got up the courage to make my third cut. I didn't make it to the next practice. I didn't even make it outside my bedroom. Then came the fourth cut ...

"I felt like somebody opened up a door and pushed me into hell."
Stevie Nicks in reference to Klonopin withdrawal.

O, God! I am a prisoner inside my own body! I can't even reach out for help because, how could I possibly explain this? If I tried, I would just sound insane, nonsensical. There are no words to describe this ... torture! Forming the words would be too distracting. I have to focus all my energy on surviving this moment. My husband is only a few feet away, and yet I've never felt so alone. No one who hasn't felt what I'm feeling could even begin to imagine this ... to understand ... "and your sufferings be sore – how sore you know not, how exquisite you know not, yea, how hard to bear you know not ... ."

My words morphed into the words of Jesus speaking to Joseph Smith.

Which suffering caused myself, even God, the greatest of all, to tremble because of pain, and to bleed at every pore, and to suffer both body and spirit—and would that I might not drink the bitter cup, and shrink—Doctrine and Covenants 19: 15,18

Ok, fine, Lord, I'll accept that if everything I have been taught is true, then you know what it's like, but no one else does.

How, in the midst of all my mental frenzy was I able to recall those words? I didn't even know if I was recalling them at the time or just creating them in my mind. They seemed real. They kept looping over and over again in my head, "how sore you know not, how exquisite you know not ... how hard to bear you know not ..." I grabbed onto those words like a drowning woman reaching for the side of a life raft floating beside her. Unable to climb in, I could barely surface from each wave as it buried my head, over and over. I held onto those words with one hand, treading water with the other as the ocean of my pain filled my lungs with more and more water. I was suffocating, every minute of every day.

I lay on the floor of my bedroom, bathed in bright yellow sunlight from the glass door and two extra windows Paul had designed into the floor plan because he knew how much I loved the sunshine. I saw the light, but I felt only darkness. My body writhed in an agony which consumed me. I imagined I looked like a parody of Harrison Ford in Indiana Jones and the Temple of Doom, where Indiana Jones, lying on a stone table, is transformed into a mindless, soulless servant of evil. His cries echo in the lonely cavern as his body and hands seize unnaturally until, finally, the transfiguration is complete. He sits up and smiles. Would my ascent from hell leave me with the same disturbingly evil grin on my face?

My old neighbor Noel called my cell phone to check up on me. It had been a while since we'd moved away. I was heartened to know she still cared and grateful for the distraction. I wanted to tell her about everything that was going on, but I didn't even know what was happening to me. All I knew was that it was painful to hold the phone up to my ear. My brain hurt from trying to interpret her words and form a reply. It hurt to feel the sun on my skin and the floor on my back. My bra straps felt like a strait jacket. Pain wasn't even the right word for it; I wouldn't have described it that way that afternoon. It was just endless, suffocating torture.

I told myself, I'm going to talk to Noel on the phone this half hour. Next half hour I'm going to walk around on the back deck. Next, I will do some stretching for the pain for 20 minutes. After that, I'll lie back down and listen to my hypnobirthing meditation for another 20 minutes. Next ...

My days and nights became a hellish marathon, spotting my next marker along the path, focusing all my energy on getting to that half hour point and the next after that until I could finally experience four or five hours of blessed relief, when I took my little bit of pill and fell into a toxic slumber. I avoided thinking of anything farther down the road. Whenever I lost focus and let my mind slip, I would begin to think about how it would be better just to lose the baby and get back on the 2 mg of Lorazepam. If I could, I would stay on it forever and never quit, ever again.

Never in my life would I have considered an abortion. In viewing the world through the lens of the gospel, the very idea of taking an innocent life was pure evil. But now I had to peer through the muddy waters of fear and pain and, to my horror, I saw abortion as a possible choice. If there were no baby, there would be no need for this agony. I could just stay on my pills and end my suffering. I caught a glimpse of the plight of so many women who, while perhaps not burning with the magnitude of flames I was in, were faced with their own crucible of choosing between the life inside of them and the life they experienced on the outside. I would never judge those women the same way again. But I had already made my choice a long time ago, at the age of eight when I was baptized and at 20 when I went through the temple. I could never take an innocent human life.

I had to stay strong; I was doing this for my baby. It would be worth it when she was born, and this was all behind me. I was a mother. Mothers made sacrifices for their children, right? There wasn't much I could do right now, but I could do that. Yes, I was in hell, but I would choose heaven.

CHAPTER 9

The Veil

When I leave this frail existence, when I lay this mortal by,
Father, Mother, may I meet you in your royal courts on high?
Then, at length, when I've completed all you sent me forth to do,
With your mutual approbation let me come and dwell with you.

HYMNS NO. 292 O MY FATHER

"I don't see a heartbeat." I'd heard those words before, with Ethan. This time was different. This was my fourth pregnancy, I was going through withdrawal, and I had Paul by my side. We were in the ER at the American Fork hospital, it was April of 2014, and I had started to bleed. I thought I might be having a miscarriage. I didn't know how I felt about the ER doctor's announcement. All I could do was try to contain the "crazy" in my brain that had become my constant companion. I could only imagine what he would think if I showed how I really felt. It was all I could do to keep from screaming, wailing, banging my head on the walls and clawing at the floor. I was like a rabid animal on the inside. But letting it out seemed more painful than keeping it inside so I stuffed the crazed benzo beast deep, deep down under the surface where I hoped it wouldn't escape. I forced out a shaky reply, hoping I didn't sound like some kind of raving lunatic.

"Do I need to deliver the baby like last time?"

"It's still early. The baby is pretty small, and you could be wrong about the date of conception, which means we might not be able to pick up a heartbeat yet." (I knew I wasn't.) "I don't want to do anything until we're completely sure this fetus isn't growing. I want you to follow up in a week with another ultrasound."

My mind tried to keep up. I had wondered many times over the past couple of months if a lot of my difficulty in withdrawing was from all the pregnancy hormones. The pelvic pain had been excruciating too. Maybe if I were no longer pregnant all this would ease up, plus, if I weren't pregnant, I wouldn't have to keep tapering. I pressed the doctor some more. "But, if the baby is dead, I don't want to keep going on with the pregnancy, wouldn't it be better just to deliver it now?" I argued. I'm sure my demeanor must have been confusing to the doctor. I didn't even understand my own logic. I just wanted to end the suffering. "I don't want to do anything drastic until we know for sure. There's still a possibility this baby could be alive," he responded.

At some point, we had already told the nurse and doctor that I was trying to get off Lorazepam. I lay there on the bed most of the time we were in the ER, with my eyes closed, breathing in and out, not daring to speak or move if I didn't have to, in case the crazy broke free when I wasn't paying attention. No one on the outside knew how much energy it took to lie there like that, silently battling the beast that raged within. I switched tactics. I asked the doctor about possibly prescribing Valium to help me with my difficult taper. I told him my husband and I had read a manual that said Valium could help people get off benzos. It said to do a program, where you keep taking the original short-acting benzo until you've slowly switched over to the longer-acting benzodiazepine. The physician told me it was definitely not recommended to take two benzos at once. "I also don't feel comfortable prescribing a category C drug when you're pregnant." "But I'm already on Lorazepam. What difference does it make which poison I'm taking?" Apparently, my frenzied logic in combination with my husband's concern and my obvious suffering was enough to overcome the ER doctor's reservations.

"What site is this? Drugs.com?" he asked. I didn't know the site. I thought the doctor might be mocking me. Paul used his phone to show him the Ashton Manual on benzo.org.uk. The doctor looked at the equivalency table provided in the first chapter of the manual, written by Professor C. Heather Ashton, DM, FRCP. I'd had great difficulty reading and understanding the manual myself, but I had gotten the gist of it. Crossover to Valium (diazepam), do a slower taper, you're not crazy. Apparently, all this agony is normal, especially considering how fast I'd been cutting and how short-acting the Ativan was. I would be prescribed enough diazepam to get me through until I could see my regular doctor. The ER doctor prescribed it to me in 10 mg and 2 mg pills. The idea was to cut the 2 mg pills and combine that with a 10 mg one to get to 13 mg, roughly the equivalent of the 1.25 mg of Lorazepam I had been taking. It was an odd prescription. I worried the pharmacy wouldn't fill it.

The pharmacy gave us no problems. In fact, the pharmacist was very interested to hear about the tapering method we were using. The next day, I felt a little better. I didn't feel good or anything. It was more like I had ascended from the ninth circle of hell to the fifth. It was a more stable agony where I no longer experienced the "drops" I felt every three to four hours as the Lorazepam broke down in my system throughout the day. When this happened, the potency diminished, and my symptoms increased until I took my evening dose. Then I would go to sleep for a few hours just to have it start all over again the next day. It was still torment on the Valium to get up, talk with someone, ride in the car, but at least now I could actually do it. I no longer felt like I might have to end my life before finishing the taper. There was hope.

We went to our follow up appointment with Dr. Scott to refill my diazepam prescription and check on the baby. It was definitely a miscarriage. It had been over a week, my hormones had dropped, and the baby wasn't growing. Dr. Scott wanted to wait for my body to miscarry naturally. Paul said he had been planning on taking the kids on a trip in a couple of weeks and asked if we could induce the miscarriage in case my body didn't deliver in time to leave town. That must have sounded like such a crazy reason to the doctor to induce a miscarriage. To be honest, it felt a bit heartless to me, but I understood. Spring break was coming up, and Paul and the kids had spent weeks worrying about mommy and the baby. He wanted to interject a happy memory into all that sorrow, start fresh, move on. I agreed to take the medication to induce a miscarriage. Maybe, if I got through this quickly, I could be well enough to make it to the gospel choir performance that weekend. I had already given up on so much of my life, having hope that I could perform with my friends again was powerful.

Dr. Scott said it would be like a bad menstrual period. Depending on how much the baby had decomposed, I may or may not see it when it came out. I went home with my prescriptions for diazepam and misoprostol. I hoped I would see something of the baby that was recognizable. But as I passed the next day in bed with contractions, all I saw were lumps of tissue and blood in the toilet. No little head or fingers or toes. It was painful, but I didn't want to take any of the medicine I'd been prescribed for the pain. I didn't need it. This wasn't the inexplicable torture of the past several weeks. This was pain I could understand. It had meaning, and that made it bearable. Residing within me on that day was clarity and a peace I hadn't experienced since before I began my taper. I even smiled when Paul brought me up some dinner that our neighbor across the street had made for our family after hearing about the miscarriage. Being a stay at home dad who excelled at his job, it was, naturally, the best chile relleno I had ever tasted.

That window of clarity closed the next day, as had the veil between life and death with yet another baby.

I had said many prayers over the past two months asking God that if it would bring me relief, to let me miscarry. I felt my prayers turn to lead on my lips. All my life, I had been taught that God is love, God is peace. You feel the Holy Ghost in that still small voice. As I prayed, I thought, how can you feel God if you can't feel love? How can he speak to you if you can't feel peace? How can you hear the whispering of the Holy Ghost when your soul is barraged night and day by a cacophony of voices, shouting at you, mocking you with your worst fears, exposing them for all the world to see?

What am I praying to? Would the God of love really let me suffer like this without any help? I'd had miraculous healings in my past, but I wasn't being healed now. Why? I needed answers, but my frenzied mind and body made it impossible to hear them. There was no way I could search the scriptures for answers; I could barely read! Right now I just needed something to hold onto, to hope for. God's presence had disappeared from my life, and I needed some evidence that he was out there somewhere. Not realizing that my now empty womb may have been a merciful answer from a loving God to my previous pleas, I prayed for the miracle of being able to sing with my friends. Crazy as it sounds, I still desperately wanted to make it to the gospel choir performance that weekend. I prayed hard.

I remembered all the times I heard people in church, bearing testimony of deeply spiritual experiences they'd had. In describing these experiences, they said that "the veil was thin," meaning transparent as if there was almost nothing separating them in that moment from the celestial realm. I'd only ever experienced something like that once in my life, in the temple. It was my first time going there for my endowment.[1] It was in Denver, Colorado, and I was 20 years old. As I completed the ceremony and passed through the temple veil to the celestial room, I suddenly had this sense that I was literally in God's presence. At that moment, someone in our group asked me if I wanted to join them in saying a prayer. The thought almost seemed absurd to me, as if bowing my head and closing my eyes would only serve to separate me from someone who I felt was right there in the room with us. If I had been alone, I would have just started talking and conversing with God like any other person.

At 35, I discovered that the transparency of the mortal veil can reveal the nature of hell as much as it does heaven. In my weakened state, there was little to defend my body and spirit from the buffetings of Satan. The shield of light, which I never realized I'd always had, that

---

1   "... temple endowment is literally a gift from God whereby he bestows sacred blessings upon you." churchofjesuschrist.org

had always protected me, had vanished. Suddenly there was this voice right next to me, constantly whispering in my ear, feeding me fear and lies. I knew they weren't true, and I knew where they were coming from, but I had no power to silence these diabolical sermons. What I am describing here is not psychosis or some hallucination. I experienced enough of those over the next year and a half of withdrawal to know the difference. This was not the effect of a frenzied mind. This was not coming from me. The mortal veil had been corroded by the chemicals I had put into my body, and I could see and hear through its perforations. It was every bit as real as my experience in the temple. Perhaps not as powerful, but just as penetrating and more than a year in duration.

Members of The Church of Jesus Christ also speak of the veil in another way. We speak of the veil of forgetfulness. This refers to "a God-given forgetfulness that blocks people's memories of the premortal existence."[2] Given the belief that we existed as spirit children with our Father in Heaven before we came to this earth, (because we are eternal beings who have and will always exist) it was necessary that we forget everything we knew before we entered mortality. If we are to learn what it means to have sorrow, joy, pleasure, pain, and faith, then we can't come to earth with an eternal perspective which sees the beginning from the end. Knowledge comes at a price.

We are born without any memory of who we are, why we're here, or what it's all about. But we are also all born with a conscience, the light of Christ, which illuminates our way back to God. I started seeking this light when I was young. I began an intense study of the

---

2   http://churchofjesuschrist.org

Book of Mormon at the age of 13. I continued nightly scripture study throughout high school while also attending seminary classes every morning before school. I continued my religious education throughout each semester of college. Like every good Latter-day Saint, I regularly attended a three-hour block of church each Sunday during which I either taught or received religious instruction.

A lifetime of religious education now became the foundation on which I built my hope. Even though I couldn't read the Bible or other scriptural canon, my injured brain could still recall what I had learned. Many times over the next two years, I would lie in bed, wishing I could study the scriptures for inspiration and comfort. Every time, despite my memory loss and severe cognitive impairment, I would recall a specific scripture that related perfectly to whatever was bothering me. At the time, it didn't strike me as communication from God. It certainly didn't "feel" that way. But in looking back, I can only consider it to be one of the many tender mercies God gave me during what would prove to be the most difficult experience of my life.

This time, as I questioned the reality of God, of everything I had ever read or been taught, I remembered 2 Nephi 2:11 from the Book of Mormon.

> 11 For it must needs be, that there is an opposition in all things. If not so, my firstborn in the wilderness, righteousness could not be brought to pass, neither wickedness, neither holiness nor misery, neither good nor bad.

My answer to my prayer wasn't a feeling of peace or light. It was a resigned acceptance of the reality of evil. It was logic in the midst of frenzy. If hell was real, then heaven was too. This was my hope. I would act on it until I was proven wrong.

I woke up the next day and rode with Paul and the kids to Salt Lake City for the gospel choir performance. I didn't know if I would be able to make it through the dress rehearsal much less the performance right after, but I decided to test my theory, to see if God was still there. I slathered essential oils all over my body in an attempt to control the pain, dizziness, and cognitive fog. By then, I had learned to compensate for the constant sense of disorientation by walking like a sailor on the deck of a ship in high seas. I probably looked like I was walking and giving birth at the same time. Lucky I was on the bottom row of the risers as I was afraid I might fall down at any moment. In between the rehearsal and the performance one of my choir mates approached me while I lay on a loveseat in the foyer of the performance hall. Paul was sitting beside me, watching over me in case I needed to make a sudden exit. "Are you nervous about the performance?" she asked. She and I had solo parts in the same song, and it was only natural that we might both be experiencing some pre-show jitters. I thought about it for a second and was surprised to find myself flatly stating "No." I didn't elaborate much, but I realized that the horror of the nightmare which had become my existence superseded any performance anxiety I might normally have had. The thought brought a wry smile to my soul. After making it through benzo withdrawals everything that used to seem scary or difficult would be a piece of cake! It was an empowering thought. I found myself clinging to it in my most desperate moments, looking forward to the transfiguration of Jocelyn from the frail, sick, weakling she had become into a powerful, fearless warrior.

I joined the rest of the cast in the green room to wait until the performance. While the other singers chatted, ate, and worked on their hair and makeup, I Iay on the floor, listening to a meditation on my phone. There was a familiar comfort to being backstage with my fellow performers, even if I was shaking from head to toe, not from fear, but from the exertion of standing and singing for so long. I was grateful to realize how socially acceptable it is to use your cellphone as an excuse to not talk to people or look them directly in the eyes, a method I would employ many times afterward. But I couldn't avoid other human beings forever, and to my relief, and distress, the audience finally arrived. It was time to perform.

I experienced what can only be described as a miracle that day. A woman who had been too sick to shower, who had become so agoraphobic she was afraid to walk out her front door, sang on stage in front of hundreds of people. Strength came to me from an unseen source like the stage lights that bathed and blinded me from above. I was still shaking, still sweating, still weak and achy from the labor pains of my induced miscarriage just a couple of days earlier, but I didn't fall down. I didn't pass out. I sang through "Hallelujah," "Purple," "Total Praise," and all the other vigorous gospel numbers, clapping shouting, smiling. I sang my solo part. Not the best performance of my life, my voice was weak, but I did it. The miracle was that I did it! I was in shock and awe as I stepped down from the risers. I knew something incredible had just happened. I tried to explain this to my family that night as we stopped by my parents' house on the way home, but un-sung words were difficult to express. I couldn't seem to make anyone understand. I didn't even understand what I was trying to explain. I just knew that something wonderful had happened.

The car sped through the darkness at 70 miles an hour on the freeway as Paul drove our family home. I covered my eyes with my hands, like a little child. I was trying to block out the view of oncoming traffic. My benzo brain made it look like every car on the road was about to slam into us at breakneck speed. Being a passenger in a vehicle was to risk death at any moment. I told myself that the fear wasn't real. Eyes still closed, I relaxed my arms, laid my head back on the headrest, and began to do some deep breathing. I focused on breathing in peace and breathing out pain. As I did, the words of The Corinthian song[2] I had sung that night echoed over and over in my mind. "Thank you, Father, for your power. It has resurrected me, over painful circumstances that my poor soul could not flee ...," over and over.

They gave me hope.

---

2   Based on 2 Corinthians 4, lyrics written by Micah Stampley

CHAPTER 10

Help

Frodo: What are we holding on to, Sam?

Sam: That there's some good in this world, Mr. Frodo. And it's
*   worth fighting for.*

THE LORD OF THE RINGS THE TWO TOWERS (2002 FILM)

I have a video on my BenzoBrains YouTube channel titled "Acceptance." It's the advice I give to people going through their benzo journeys that I wish I'd had when starting mine. This was a video I made two years after finishing my 15-month taper off Lorazepam and diazepam. It expounds on the most frequent advice I give to desperate benzo victims coming to me for help, which is to "accept, accept, accept, distract, distract, distract." It's the best advice I can give anyone who has to deal with unbearable circumstances over which they have no control. It's what I was told by a volunteer in the support group I was in when I was desperate for help.

It's hard to accept that your whole world has changed when you don't have the ability to look down on your life from above and see it for what it really is. When the whole world is telling you this should only take a few weeks and that it's just a matter of willpower and positive thinking, you question the reality of your own suffering. It's easier to accept the labels of lazy, malingering, insane, or weak than to come to the realization that you have suddenly become someone with a severe disability. In my "Acceptance" video, I try to be the friend I wish I'd had when I was in withdrawal: "I give you permission to go to the doctor and fill out one of those forms that you take to the DMV so you can get a handicapped placard and park in the handicapped parking at the grocery store. Just because people can't see your disability, because it's at a cellular level, that doesn't make it any less real." I needed someone to tell me that during the spring of 2014.

After the gospel choir performance, Paul single-handedly planned, packed, and drove our family to California for our first trip ever to Disneyland. Business had suddenly taken off, and he decided to use the extra income to splurge on a hotel right next to the park so I could be with our family and also retire to the hotel as easily as possible. We ordered room service to avoid the extra effort of traveling to restaurants or preparing our own food. The surface of my memories of this trip are all happy. I see reflections of the beautiful bright hotel room with its crisp white down comforters and oversized feather pillows. It looks out directly over Paradise Pier so we can watch the world of color water show from our window at night. I feel the excitement of the children at being greeted by Goofy in the hotel lobby and my gratitude for the kindness shown to my little ones, for the extra attention they receive as first-time visitors. There's an amnesia that follows trauma. It anesthetizes the memory of pain. I consider that to be a gift of grace, a heavenly filter that covers the lens of our minds and creates a safe place for us in which to heal.

I now have the strength to remove the gauze of selective memory and look at the scars that remain. I see myself, looking out the passenger window as we drive to California, observing the passing desert landscape that separates the Rocky Mountains from the lush California coast. My heart aches as I recall how we had to stop and stay at Paul's parents' in Las Vegas. Even that five-hour drive required several pit stops so I could slowly unbend my body and attempt to walk off the physical pain and madness, the effects of sitting still for too long. The children are in the back watching movies on the TV headrests Paul installed in the car before we left. I don't dare speak. I might break if I do. Paul has no idea what traveling in a car in my condition is doing to me. Hour by hour, it keeps getting worse and worse. Halfway through the trip, I surface from the darkness of my torment and lift my eyes to the sky to say a silent prayer. "Please, Father, let me die." I have no energy to put any more words together into a rational statement. I exhale my prayer and sink back under the rolling waves of darkness.

We arrive at the hotel the next day, and I wait in the lobby with the kids and the luggage, as Paul checks us in. I try not to make eye contact with anyone and hope that my 3- and 7-year-olds don't require any discipline from me as I don't have the cognitive ability to engage in creative parenting. Paul and the kids want to go to the beach. I want to go with them; if I could only nap first! I hadn't been able to do more than lie in a fitful state of rest since starting my taper. Oh, I would fall asleep around midnight, after taking my diazepam, but I awoke every single morning at 5:30 a.m. to my heart pounding, sweating through the sheets, and my bowels in such state that I had to make a mad dash through the darkness to the toilet. That was my alarm clock. There was no going back to bed after that. I was holding for now at 13 mg of diazepam until I felt strong enough to continue the withdrawal process.

I figured the day I could lie down and relax enough to fall asleep without taking a pill, would be a significant sign that healing was taking place, and I could go back to tapering.

The next morning I walked across the street with my family and into the happiest place on earth. I tried to feel something other than guilt as my kids were greeted by theme park characters and classic Disney soundtracks. I waited in line, debating whether or not I could handle Toy Story Mania for my kids' sake. I don't know how, but somehow, I managed to get on a couple of rides by keeping my eyes closed and holding my head in my hands to keep it from jerking back and forth. I even started to feel better for a little bit as we stood in line, absorbing the sunlight through my skin and breathing in the moist coastal air. There was enough anonymity in the crowd that I didn't feel too conspicuous and the jumble of voices, machinery, and music blended together into white noise. Maybe this is what it means to "stabilize," the thing people on the BenzoBuddies forum describe when discussing how to begin a taper program. It's important to stabilize on the right medication and the right dose before making any cuts, especially if you've already attempted a fast reduction. I was hoping to stabilize before resuming my taper. I assumed "stable" meant I would get to a point where I felt kind of normal again.

This wasn't normal. It was what's known as a good window, a natural fluctuation in the process of healing from this kind of injury to the nervous system. Good times are referred to as windows and especially bad times are called waves. I didn't know this was a window, but it was something hopeful. I was doing it. Maybe this really is about mind over matter I told myself. Then it hit, right after lunch. I couldn't take one more step. I needed to get back to the hotel immediately. Paul installed an app on our phones so I could see exactly where they were at any given moment; that way, I would still feel like a part of things. Then he gave me instructions on what to do, how to ride the rail back to the entrance and make my way back to the hotel. It was difficult to remember, even though I had him repeat it to me several times. How could I possibly make it all the way back to our room when I no longer had the strength to stand? I wanted to ask him to take me back, but I didn't want to make the family sacrifice that much time out of their fun day.

I tried to visualize my path home. "Just keep swimming." Dory from *Finding Nemo* became my cheerleader ... "just keep swimming, just keep swimming, what do we do we swim ...," I repeated the words over and over as I put one foot in front of the other. I tried to think of how I could ask the person standing next to me on the train for help, but what would I say? "Can you please carry me back to my hotel room?" Somehow I made it to the lobby. "Ok, just push the elevator button, you're almost there," I told myself. Waiting for the elevator doors to open seemed like weeks. They finally parted. I walked in as calmly as I could and rode up to what I hoped was the right floor. I stepped out into the hallway and tried to decipher which direction the numbers on the signs were directing me to walk. Paul had told me our room number, but I couldn't retain the sequence of numbers in my head. I honestly think it was just luck and divine guidance that led me to the right room. I put the key card into the slot and made the world's slowest dash to the queen-sized bed. I made one last effort to sit up and pull back the covers so I could slide underneath them. I was safe.

If I could have cried, I would have, but I couldn't. I wanted to cry for the anguish I felt at not being able to be with my family, for the humiliation of being so pathetic that the journey from the park to my hotel room felt like a Herculean endeavor. I wanted to shed tears of relief for having made it anyway, but no tears came. You'd think that with all this pain and sorrow, I would have been crying all the time, but tears are a luxury reserved for people who get to feel real emotions. My soul had been wrung dry, and my tears had evaporated in the crucible I'd been living in the past two months. No amount of writhing and groaning could produce a single tear. No matter how hard I tried. So I just closed my eyes and focused on the sterile softness of the sheets.

I awoke to an orange-hued light saturating my hotel room. I had slept. It was a few hours later than when I had lain down, and the sun was entering the last leg of its journey west across the sky. It was a miracle! I had honestly believed I might never be able to fall asleep without drugs again. I felt a surge of gratitude as I lay there, not wanting to move and risk disturbing the peace I felt in that moment. I wanted to see my family, though, so I got up and called Paul on his cell phone to arrange to meet with him and the kids. I made it until the early evening. The trip back to the hotel was made easier by the presence of my husband and kids. Paul got Nathaniel and Lucy ready for bed. Then they watched the *World of Color* in their pajamas from our window as I lay in bed. My strength was gone, but I had made it. Tomorrow I might be able to go half a day again, then rest and go another half day. This could work.

The next morning I didn't even make it into the park. I sat down on a bench and told Paul that if he wanted me to join them, he would need to find a wheelchair. He was really upset. We were already later than he had anticipated and he didn't want to lose any more time. My husband went off in the direction of the main entrance while I waited with the kids, I think. I don't remember who was with me. I don't remember him bringing the electric wheelchair. All I remember is that we had strict instructions not to allow anyone to sit in my lap, or we would lose wheelchair privileges. Paul had to carry Lucy on his back as we traveled through the park that day.

We had no idea that being in a wheelchair at Disneyland had its advantages. You got to go to the front of the line at every ride so the workers could admit you and everyone in your party through a special wheelchair accessible entrance. That brightened Paul's day. I didn't feel so guilty about being such a burden after that. But it was hard not to allow Lucy to sit in my lap, especially when Paul took Nathaniel to a ride that was too big for someone her age. He asked me to wait while they went to a different area of the park. We had been left by a splash pad and, since it was warm, Lucy could play in the water until daddy and Nano came back. She happily handed me her sandals and made her way to the mini water fountains. A park attendant approached me as I sat in my chair and told me that my child had to keep her shoes on, or we would be asked to leave. I called Lucy over to me, and weakly explained that she needed her shoes on. She began to get angry as I tried to put her shoes back on her feet. She screamed as I tried to hold her back from running off with bare feet. I didn't know what to do or what to say. If I let her go, would the guy try to kick us out? Would I get kicked out of my chair if I tried to hold her in my lap? I couldn't come up with a reasonable solution.

Lucy never threw fits. I had read *The Happiest Toddler on the Block* back when Nathaniel was about her age, and I knew how to nip a fit right in the bud before it exploded. I used to be supermom. Why couldn't I figure out how to do something as simple as getting my daughter to wear her sandals? She refused to calm down, and I was too afraid even to attempt to reason with her in front of all those people. I just held Lucy's hand tight to keep her from running and silently begged for Paul to get back as soon as possible.

Other kids began to play without their shoes on. Nobody said anything to them, but it was too late for us. Lucy was frantic. I kept calling Paul's cell, trying to listen through the screaming only to hear his voicemail pick up the call. What was taking so long?! Finally a lady approached me and asked me if I needed help. Her act of compassion primed the pump and I felt tears welling up inside me. I said as little as possible because I knew if I said too much I might start sobbing uncontrollably. After weeks of not being able to cry, this was an inconvenient moment to start. And really, how do you ask for help when you don't have a name for what's wrong? I managed to say something about my husband being somewhere else without any tears. The well was still too dry. I think she tried to help with Lucy after that. I don't remember.

Finally, they came back. I was furious. I wanted to yell at my husband for leaving me there, but I was too weak and scared to rail at him. Paul reminded me that he had explained how to get to where he was before he left. It wasn't that far, but that didn't matter. He might as well have given me instructions on how to walk to the moon. I had been stranded. I wanted to make him understand that it wasn't ok to leave me like that, to tell him I wasn't the person he thought I was anymore. But I couldn't. Instead, I made a half-hearted complaint about the employee being a jerk and then made Paul promise to only get on rides that Lucy could go on for the rest of the day. I pretended not to be furious. At one point, I even obligingly got out of my wheelchair so Paul could take pictures of the kids and me.

"Smile," Paul instructed, and as he did, I saw myself holding our lifeless baby in a coarse medical blanket in the hospital room. "Smile," Paul had pleaded as he used the disposable camera Dottie had given to us. Why do I need to smile? Why can't he just take a picture of what's really going on? Why am I being asked to fake an emotion that's totally inappropriate for this situation? I did my best for his sake, though. I didn't look like I was smiling in the hospital photograph, more like a weird, ugly cry. It's easier to fake a smile when you can't cry. Our pictures from Disneyland 2014 were a little too convincing.

When we got back to Utah, I pleaded for help from my family.[1] I sent out texts, begging for someone to come take the kids for an afternoon or a weekend, just to get them out of the house, so they wouldn't have to be around their sick mom all day. Their dad needed a break, and I needed relief from the constant guilt I felt at failing to be the mother my children needed every minute of the day. I wanted my family and friends to rally around me and offer me the kind of compassion and help my neighbor with breast cancer down the street was getting. But they didn't see me like someone with an illness as painful and debilitating as someone going through chemo. My parents told Paul I just needed to get out of the house and get outside my head. But you can't just get out of your head when you're being poisoned, whether by chemo or benzos, because it's not "in your head" that's the problem. Disabled by physical and emotional suffering, I was confined to my

---

1   As I heal I realize how skewed my perception of my loved ones was during that time. This is part of the nature of a benzodiazepine injury and not an uncommon effect. It's likely my family reached out in many ways that I did not perceive or that were misinterpreted. I attempt to be true to what I experienced during that time in my writing.

room and Nathaniel and Lucy were mostly left to fend for themselves whenever Paul wasn't home. I felt abandoned, and my heart ached for my children. I mourned for my husband. The only other thing I could think to do for my family was to be as little a burden as possible. I would try not to talk too much about my symptoms and encourage Paul and the kids to get out of the house often.

We ended up hiring a friend I'd sung with in the gospel choir to help with the kids and household chores, like Alice from the *Brady Bunch*. Nyrie was young, newly married, and working part-time cleaning hospitals while she pursued singing gigs on the side. Both she and her husband had been prescribed various psychiatric medications over the years to help with depression, anxiety, and ADHD. She knew what it was to be cognitively disabled to some degree and to feel awkward and misunderstood. We told her the position would only be part-time for the spring and summer until the kids went back to school. Surely by then, I would start to get better. Nyrie was happy to help us out. This trendy millennial with closely coiffed black hair and pale skin (indicative of a mixed Brazilian/Caucasian heritage) became my angel of mercy. She didn't care that I wasn't the old me because she never really knew the old me. I would apologize for not being a very good conversationalist, for being so slow and sad all the time. She would just shrug and tell me she liked me the way I was. When I could no longer put on a brave face and a positive attitude, when the tears (or lack thereof) would overwhelm me as I lay, incapacitated in bed, Nyrie would sit beside me and tenderly hold my hand as I washed her with a flood of worries and sorrows, most of which probably sounded nonsensical. She never judged me. She just listened. She was compassionate, and that was all I needed.

My sister was getting married in May, and both she and my mother were busy making preparations. Despite this, my mom would occasionally make the trip down from Sandy after work to help out. Mom has always had severe anxiety, and my situation really stressed her out. I could feel her frustration when she walked through the door, and it was too much for me to handle. I would go upstairs to avoid watching her go into hyper mode. Instead of taking the kids to the park or sitting next to me and holding my hand, mom would start cleaning like mad. I could feel her resentment towards me as I cowered in my room. I knew she was angry at me for not talking to her, but I didn't know how else to ask for help or how to explain what was going on. I was angry at her for not understanding. I was angry at everyone. My family had practically ignored me during the miscarriage. Only my mom and my soon-to-be brother-in-law texted me their condolences. None of them accepted my invitation to attend the gospel choir performance, but they all knew I stood and sang on stage for over an hour. Now they had just seen me standing and smiling at Disneyland. "Why should they go out of their way to accommodate me?" I thought. My family saw me go through Cymbalta withdrawal. They knew I acted weird and anxious, but it wasn't a big deal. I guess they think it's the same thing this time, especially after my Disneyland trip. "I wish they could spend just five minutes in my body! They would go running to the ER, terrified they were dying. Then they would understand." Darker thoughts than these plagued me every time my mom came over. It was a relief when she left.

May came, and I was still holding, waiting for that magical stabilization to happen. I learned more about how to taper using compounds and homemade suspensions. The liquid valium I asked Dr.

Scott to prescribe me made me feel even worse. I went back on the pills. Things weren't getting any better than the first day I'd switched to diazepam. I guessed this was as good as it was going to get. I decided to begin my micro taper after my sister's wedding.

Not being able to eat much, and frequent trips to the bathroom did have their advantages. I continued to lose weight, and my stomach got smaller and smaller. I look at the pictures of my sister's wedding, and I see a woman with a teeny waist and bloated hands and face, symptoms of dehydration. I wish I could say I remember my sister's sealing in the temple. I'd like to have the image of Michelle kneeling there across the altar from her husband, beautifully arrayed in white and say that I remember the feeling in the room as the sealer spoke words of eternal significance to them. But I don't. I remember being outside, taking pictures and then, miraculously once again being able to nap at my brother's house in between the temple ceremony and the reception. I remember having another good window that evening that made it possible for me to fake happiness enough to get by without casting a shadow on her special day. At least, I hope that's what I did.

I don't know why God helped me to have these miraculous windows on certain occasions. One might say, "well, it's about mind over matter, you wanted it bad enough, so you did it." But there were so many other times when I desired just as desperately to be well enough to go somewhere, have a conversation, fake my way through an event, and I wasn't capable. It wasn't just about will power. There were far more times when I couldn't than when I could. It seems that my miracles were usually more for the benefit of others than for myself. In fact, if anything, my good windows only served to further convince those around me that my situation was not so dire as I claimed.

That's the wicked nature of this illness. As the different systems in your body attempt to balance out as you heal, you have immense fluctuations in symptoms and ability. One day, you might be able to go outside and weed the garden, and the next, you are practically or literally catatonic on the floor. It's very hard to convince others to help you when what they see looks like a woman cherry-picking her disability day by day. I couldn't explain it myself. One day, I found a fantastic blog written by a survivor on the benzo support forum. It described how our fluctuating symptoms were manifestations of a central nervous system that was shutting down and reloading various programs, much like rebooting a computer. Finally, I had a narrative that made sense! I asked Paul to help me print out several copies and hand them out to family members at our next birthday dinner.

In my family, every time someone has a birthday, my mom will cook them a special dinner and invite everyone over. This must have been my nephew's special dinner. Knowing him, he asked for sopapillas, green chile, spanish rice, and beans. I picked at my food and waited until we were cleaning up to give everyone the handout. I told them it explained what I was going through and asked them to read it. A few weeks later, I asked some of them if they had looked at it. Only mom had, but when I asked what she thought of it, she gave me a nonchalant shrug accompanied by a similar verbal response. I was heartbroken. I thought this explanation would be the key to unlocking their hearts and minds, granting me access to the love and understanding I so desperately needed. But that wouldn't happen for a long time.

I was Gregor Samsa in *The Metamorphosis*. I had become a great ugly beetle who was not only useless but had become an awkward annoyance to everyone else. I hadn't learned to accept my new disconcerting exoskeleton. I was still waiting to change back. As time went on, I learned that accepting this change in myself precipitated any ability to truly seek help from others. I eventually developed a whole new way of communicating with people so they could look past the nauseating outer shell and see the fragile bits of me that still existed underneath. This took time, though, and it wasn't something I could do during the worst of my withdrawal. I tried, but the labor of trying to communicate and failing over and over made me weary and even more depressed. It was easier to pretend everything was normal, even though I couldn't come close to successfully feigning normalcy. I knew how weird I seemed to everyone else. But that weird was me doing my best to contain the crazy. You try wrestling with a rabid beast the size of Mount Everest while having a conversation about the weather and see how normal you come off.

I remember one spring day, before the wedding, I decided to go outside to get some sunlight. I grabbed the big red furry blanket my grandma Lucy had made and picked the sunniest patch on the lawn to sit on as it was an unusually cold day. I just wanted to feel some sunlight on my face and breathe something other than the stale air in my bedroom. Paul had been working hard to finish the basement in our home, so my sister and her husband could move in downstairs. The dust and noise had become unbearable enough to motivate me to overcome my agoraphobia and go outside in the day time. I happened to be sitting by the sidewalk at the corner of our white picket fence. Some neighbors walked by, a couple who only a few months ago had gone on a double date with Paul and me to a Brian Regan concert.

I must have looked a sight, wrapped in that blanket, sitting a few feet away from the road for all the neighborhood to see. My frizzy hair unkempt, the crazed expression on my pale face accentuated my sunken eyes as I stared at nothing in the distance. As they stopped to check on me, they offered an awkward "Hi." They asked if I was feeling ok. I considered saying something. Then I imagined my friends being overwhelmed by the vision of eternity they might see were I to open my mouth and they take a peek inside, like the Hindu god Vishnu. I didn't want to expose them to the endless black coldness of the universe I held inside me, so I gave them a half-smile and said that I just wasn't feeling very well. They politely wished me well and continued on their way.

How do you ask people to help you when you're afraid of yourself? How do you reach out to others when you're separated from them by an endless void of suffering? There are so many seemingly unanswerable questions when one is in unbearable pain. There are countless people in this world right now who are incapacitated by their suffering. The irony of this tragedy is that those most in need of help are the least able to seek it out. Yet everyone needs an advocate. How often have you or I asked for mercy, even when we weren't sure we deserved it? When is it ever fair for someone to ask the people around her to do more for her than she can do for them? But it happens all the time. How many of us realize how desperate we really are, how blessed we have been, how grateful we should be for the goodness of God reflected in those around us?

I created my YouTube channel to be the advocate I wished I'd had. I receive messages on my videos almost daily from viewers, messages like:

"Thank you for a truly inspiring video. You gave me so much hope when I really needed it."

And: "It's so great to have you as a guide through all this hell. Can't find the words to thank you enough."

"I wonder," one viewer responded on my video for loved ones of benzo victims, "if you realize what a gift your videos are to all of us."

Another said: "Bless you! My sister has been going through this withdrawal for a year and we haven't even known what it was. She has been in and out of the psych ward four times in a year. ...Thank you so much for this video.! I'm doing all these things but have been feeling so horrible and sad that I am not doing enough! I can't fix it!!! You made me feel like what I am doing matters even though it doesn't fix the problem. And that gives me some peace, thank you!"

I think that's what it means when Jesus says, "blessed are the poor in spirit for theirs is the kingdom of heaven." The people who come to my channel are truly poor in spirit, but that poverty has the potential to become a wealth of immeasurable value "where neither moth nor rust doth corrupt, and where thieves do not break through nor steal."

I'm no savior, but I do see his hand in my advocacy work. I see it in the lives of those who come to me for help. Gratitude is the most common response they have, a fingerprint of his intervening grace. Sure, there are those who get angry at me, try to argue with me or dismiss me. But most of the people who come to my channel have been hollowed out, their pride extinguished. They know they are infinitely incapable of making their case to the world and any help in doing so is infinitely appreciated. Jesus said:

Listen to him who is the advocate with the Father, who is pleading your cause before him—

Saying: Father, behold the sufferings and death of him who did no sin, in whom thou wast well pleased; behold the blood of thy Son which was shed, the blood of him whom thou gavest that thyself might be glorified; Wherefore, Father, spare these my brethren that believe on my name, that they may come unto me and have everlasting life.

Doctrine & Covenants 45: 3-5

After going through benzo withdrawal, many people find their priorities change. Like me, their lives are never the same again.

And that's not necessarily a bad thing.

CHAPTER 11

Gods in Embryo

Sometimes our light goes out but is blown again into flame by an encounter with another human being. Each of us owes the deepest thanks to those who have rekindled this light.

ALBERT SCHWEITZER

The two most comforting words anyone can hear are "I understand." It's what the son of God can say to every person who has ever lived because he has felt their pain. Even though he lived a perfect life, he chose to subject himself to every horrible experience in mortality that comes from sin, sickness, and a corrupted world. Through no fault of his own, he experienced infinite suffering in the Garden of Gethsemane so that he could help us, so he would know how to comfort us, so he could truly love us. I don't totally understand what Jehovah experienced that day in the garden of olive trees, but I do know what endless and eternal suffering feels like.

There is no time in the infinite loop of internal tortures when you are a prisoner inside your own mind and body. Every minute of what is known as acute benzo withdrawal syndrome is like an R-rated horror film version of *Groundhog Day*. It's hard for those looking in from the outside to know what to do for someone in that situation.

Sometimes neighbors and friends would make comments like, "when I had insomnia, I did this ..." which is great except, insomnia wasn't my problem. It was merely one of the 50 plus symptoms I experienced on any given day and low on my list of ones that were most worrisome. Or like my well-intentioned acupuncturist who, at our appointment on Halloween Day 2014 cheerfully inquired, "Are you being a scarecrow for Halloween?" He honestly didn't realize that my look was an unintentional byproduct of severe weight loss coupled with the inability to fix my frizzy, bleached, straw-colored hair or wear anything tighter than a loose-fitting flannel shirt and linen pants. I can laugh about these things now. But at the time it was just another blow to an already degrading experience. I knew I looked awful with my sunken, glassy eyes, but at least my skin was clear, so I didn't have to worry about makeup. I'd spent many years well into adulthood dealing with acne, not severe but just annoying enough to make me self-conscious. Clear skin was a blessing for which I was grateful, even if my hair was falling out by the handful. I thought about movies and images I'd seen of Japanese women who'd been exposed to radiation from atomic bombs. One woman screamed while looking at a clump of hair she had just pulled from her head. I might have done the same, but what was the point of screaming? I'd have sacrificed my whole head of hair if it meant the suffering would stop.

I've had many people express sympathy to me in my life when I've gone through terrible things. Friends shared their sorrow for me when I lost my baby. Acquaintances took pity on me and stepped in when I could not care for my children after being disabled by psych meds. The compassion my friends and neighbors had for me was meaningful and very much needed. But there's something different about connecting with someone who has been there, who knows exactly what it feels like to walk where you have walked. It's not that the tears of people who, for instance, haven't lost a baby are any less real, it's just that those who have lost a child know what to say. They know exactly what they can do to help. But above all, I know they know what it feels like, and that makes one feel less like an object of pity alone on an island of suffering and more like part of the shared human experience.

There's a bond that connects us to others in tragedy. The blazing furnace of suffering is the great equalizer. Mists of race, wealth, gender, and religion that obscure our understanding dissipate before its intense heat and, perhaps for the first time, we can truly see the person standing in front of us.

In early May of 2014, I was still trying to figure out how to taper as slowly from the diazepam as the Ashton Manual recommends. I really didn't like the way this new benzo made me feel, but it was better than the "drops" I experienced throughout the day on the Lorazepam. However, cutting pieces off of those pills was still too drastic a reduction and would be too jarring to my system. The liquid version wasn't an option; it made me even worse. None of the doctors I reached out to knew what to do. The local detox facility said they couldn't help me. I was stuck. In his methodical way of approaching any problem, Paul did some research and found several online support groups for people going through benzo withdrawal. He talked with me about the possibility of reaching out to one of them for help. I recoiled from the idea. Some of this was just irrational fear due to my altered brain chemistry. But I think some of it was also related to the stigma of addiction and withdrawal. It was already difficult enough wresting the sympathy I needed from friends and family. Besides, I wasn't an addict. I didn't want to be part of a group of people who had cravings for a drug that I wanted nothing more than to get off of. I couldn't relate to people who used benzos irresponsibly when I had only ever taken them as prescribed.

It wasn't until later in May, when my father-in-law visited with me, that I changed my mind. I knew Dan had been in a terrible car accident when Paul was 15 years old. The impact of both the seatbelt strap and hitting the steering wheel broke his sternum in three places. His brain was injured too. You can't see the damage, but it's there, inside his skull. It's called a TBI, traumatic brain injury. Dan and Delores have related to me at times how difficult it has been to deal with this injury because people have difficulty understanding such a complex problem, especially when it can't be seen. I could relate to that.

Being a quiet and reserved man, Dan and I had rarely had intimate conversations. Looking back, my naturally boisterous personality was probably a bit much for him to endure at times. Now though, I was no longer one to dominate a conversation or even to speak at all for that matter. Dan came up from the downstairs office and sat in a chair across from the couch on which I was resting. He started telling me about his accident, relating it to me in greater detail than ever before. He told me how much he hated seeing the psychiatrist who would ask him questions like, "Are you having any thoughts about harming yourself? How would you do it?" These questions turned Dan's mind in directions he didn't want to go. He was already dealing with feelings of sadness and hopelessness caused by the constant pain and inability to function after his accident. But suicide wasn't even a consideration until the psychiatrist brought it up. His doctor would then "tweak" the various medications he'd been prescribing Dan and send him on his way.

Along with the physical and psychological battles, my father-in-law and his wife spent the next four and a half years after his accident battling with their insurance company to cover his medical expenses. It turned into a brutal legal battle that literally added insult to his injury. According to Dan, the one place that gave him hope was the support group. There he could see how other people were doing, what similar struggles they were going through, and how their marriages were just as tenuous as his own. It was through his support group that Dan learned about supplements that could manage his pain better than the opiates he'd been prescribed. He also learned about herbal remedies he could use in place of psychiatric drugs.

Ironically, it wasn't until my father-in-law saw me go through this experience that he realized how much the medications he had been prescribed at the time, increased the severity of his condition. For some reason, when somebody's brain is bludgeoned, doctors find it logical to introduce it to chemical cocktails. Dan couldn't even remember the names of all the drugs he had been taking, but he knew that some were antidepressants, opiates, and tranquilizers. By the time the court case was finally settled, most of the money had run out. My in-laws didn't have the means to pay for Dan's continuing medical treatment, and that was probably a blessing in disguise. He said he felt better ditching the psychiatrist and going for little walks in the mornings. Dan used what he had been learning about herbs to wean himself rapidly off all his medications. Eventually, he was able to walk for miles each day after dropping Paul off at his early morning seminary class. Then, somehow, Paul's Dad would manage to take his son to school, drive himself to vocational rehabilitation to be assessed, and do menial labor like assembling and packaging garden twirlers. After all that, he would come home and go straight to bed.

Dan found it difficult to interact with his family during those years of recovery. His personality had completely changed. His wife was often at her wit's end. She was caring for the two boys they still had at home, teaching piano, and making ends meet without her husband's income. It was a dark time in his family's history, and I could see that it was painful for my father-in-law to discuss.

But after he healed from the medications, the broken sternum, the brain trauma, and the degrading lawsuit, Dan found ways to be whole again. He implemented mindfulness techniques to deal with the chronic pain and found alternative practitioners to help him manage the effects of his TBI. Neuropsychological testing helped my father-in-law learn how to recognize his limitations and organize tasks in a way that worked around his brain injury. Once a successful accountant, Dan now had brain fatigue, which kept him from putting in a full workday. Accepting this, he found ways to work part-time consistently in the years following his accident.

I knew things still weren't easy for this 65-year-old man and yet, I saw before me someone who tried, someone who, despite the odds, had made it through to the other side, and that gave me hope. Dan's story helped me move past my fears and reach out for the peer support I so desperately needed. I got online that night and signed on to benzobuddies.org. Navigating an online web forum was completely foreign to me, though, and in my mental confusion, it was impossible for me to learn. I reluctantly decided to forgo the anonymity of the forum and just join one of the Facebook groups I had seen pop up in my searches.

How I wish I had joined sooner! I got immediate responses to questions I'd been asking the doctors for months. I found that I was not alone in taking a low dose as prescribed; in fact, I wasn't even in the minority! Almost everyone there had a story similar to mine. I learned how to implement a tapering strategy using my pills known as liquid titration, something I could have easily done with the Ativan had I known sooner. I learned there were other women in the group who had also had miscarriages while tapering Lorazepam too quickly. They private messaged me, and we became close friends. One day, after waking up from a nap, I posted:

> *K just have to get this off my chest — one of my worst sxs (side effects) I experience is when I'm groggy or coming out of a nap, I could totally be talking to my kids or husband and then suddenly it's like something shuts off. It's like I went to sleep, but I can hear and am aware of what's going on around me, even see a little. For the life of me, I can't move! I can't come out of it, and it's terrifying! The only thing I can control is my breathing, and so I make moaning noises, and if someone is around they'll shake me out of it, but if I don't keep my mind going, I'll slip right back. Is this some form of dp/dr (depersonalization /derealization).[1]*

The answers came immediately.

Gary — it sounds like withdrawal induced sleep paralysis.

---

[1]   The feeling that you're observing yourself from outside your body or you have a sense that things around you aren't real, or both. Mayoclinic.org I experience these as a disconnect from the physical world and myself. It felt like I was constantly trying to see, hear, talk and move through mud.

Stacey — I used to get that all the time at the beginning of my taper. I promise as you get lower it goes away.

I was told to google sleep paralysis. I did and discovered that I could do little tricks to kick myself out of it like scrunching my face or wiggling my big toe. It was still scary, and it went on for more than a year, but now that I had a name for that symptom, it wasn't quite as terrifying. It was a real thing, it was a normal part of withdrawal, and it would go away. That's all I needed to hear.

I found faces I could relate to on YouTube as well. It made me feel less lonely watching real people talk about their own experiences in going through this horror. It was comforting to hear them put into words what I couldn't express myself. "Yes!" I would say as I watched one man speak in his video about looking into a mirror and seeing unrecognizable, glassy, soulless eyes staring back at him, "that's exactly how I feel." I clung to the words of a young woman named Ally, who explained all the various symptoms she and I experienced on any given day:

Vertigo/dizziness
twitching
anhedonia (inability to experience pleasure)
depersonalization (feeling like you are outside your body)
derealization (feeling like you're experiencing the world through a
    fishbowl, like trying to breathe through mud)
sensitivity to heat/cold
numbness
burning sensations of the face and scalp

nausea and poor appetite

looping/paranoid thoughts

suicidality

fear/terror

tinnitus

blurry vision/eye floaters

teeth pain

weight loss

painful, rock hard stomach bloating (benzo belly)

sensitivity to chemicals and foods

sensitivity to sound and light

shortness of breath

heart palpitations

feeling like you're going to blackout every time you stand up (postural orthostatic tachycardia syndrome)

cog fog

pain in the joints, muscles skin, eyes

rage

insomnia

rebound dreaming (vivid dreams usually nightmarish)

The list goes on and on, and most symptoms are experienced all together every day. But the point really wasn't how many symptoms Ally had to deal with on any given day. The point was that no one recognized them as benzo withdrawal syndrome. The doctors said it couldn't all be from the few short weeks she had been on Xanax, and all the testing she had undergone proved useless. I could relate to that. Ally was intelligent, lovely, well-spoken, and the only thing she could do was to tell her story in the hope that it might help someone else. She was a beacon in the darkness for me; she had given me a voice. Ally was me.

When I found out she was lesbian, I realized that didn't change how I felt about her. I hadn't had much of an opportunity to really get to know many people who were openly LGBTQ before my entry into the world of social media. Even though we had never met face to face, I loved Ally. She was just one of many people from all walks of life with whom I developed a friendship. Most of them were like me in that they had never abused their benzodiazepine. But some were or had been addicts. It didn't matter. I relied on them as much as they relied on me. When I saw how easy it is to self-medicate when doctor after doctor is unable or unwilling to help, I realized that could have been me. How true the old adage is "there but for the grace of God go I."

Some of my new friends were almost militantly atheist. I could honestly understand why, and it didn't change how I felt about them. I was struggling with my own faith, but I still hoped God was there, and they were no less compassionate than the rest, their stories no less heartbreaking. Because of these friendships, I considered, perhaps, for the first time in my life, political and philosophical ideologies which, prior to benzos, I would have outright dismissed. How unthreatening are ideas when you care more about the person to which they belong! It reminds me of the concept of Zion, which has many definitions. One of them is many people being of one heart and one mind. In church, we're always talking about building up or establishing Zion on the earth. Zion can be physical and spiritual, but the goal is to do everything we can to create an ideal society through our churches, communities, and families.

To my mind, Zion was this perfect place where nobody had any problems. But now I think Zion is a place where people still struggle, but those hardships are shared by everyone. Sufferers are embraced, understood, and loved. Everyone united in heart may eliminate many worldly problems, but even when unavoidable challenges arise, the burden is made lighter because everyone shares the load. I saw evidence of this in both my online and local communities.

A common statement you hear in the support groups is, "I wouldn't wish this on my worst enemy." That's not a hollow statement. We really can't imagine knowingly inflicting such horrors on another human being, no matter what suffering they themselves may have perpetuated. This leads to some very sick and weak people spending their precious energy warning, educating, and encouraging others. There's no going back in time to prevent this from happening to us. But maybe, just maybe, we can stop it from happening to our neighbor, our daughter, or our boyfriend. If not, then at least we could ease the burdens on those who had come looking for relief. Saving someone from making the same mistakes we did, whether it was with tapering or in communicating with their doctor, was a huge victory. We were unified in our weakness, and that made us deeply invested in strengthening one another. One person's success or failure belonged to us all. I can't imagine anything more Zion-like than that!

I had a sense now and then of how I was seeing the best in humanity displayed in the worst of circumstances, and it gave me hope. I was and will always be grateful to those people who responded with compassion and empathy to my questions and fears, even though I know I must have been difficult to handle. Benzo people aren't always the easiest people to talk to or comfort. Our minds don't work the same as a healthy person's. The benzo beast rears its ugly head in many different ways, one of which is known as benzo rage. This uncontrollable, irrational anger can be frightening for both the one displaying it and whoever is on the receiving end. In our family, the receiver was usually my husband. I'm a small woman, and he's a large man, so luckily, I wasn't physically threatening to him. Still, I cringe when I think back to the night when, in the heat of the moment, I took the large glass jar I had been holding and chucked it at Paul's head, having every intention of hitting him square in the face. I wasn't standing more than two feet from my husband, but because my coordination was so abysmal at the time, I blessedly missed his head, breaking the jar on the wall behind him instead. We can laugh now about how weak and ridiculous I was at the time. But that's not always the case in every relationship. Sometimes the person on the receiving end is a woman, and it's a man who is possessed by the benzo beast. Those situations aren't so funny.

Basically, this illness makes benzo victims as unloveable and un-relatable as possible. An invisible illness caused by a few doses of medication with symptoms that change from day to day, sometimes hour by hour? Who would even believe such a thing, much less upend their lives to accommodate someone who looks like they're either crazy or going through heroin withdrawal? But there are angels who exist in human form. They believe us. They save us from ourselves.

As the summer came to an end, I struggled to imagine how I could possibly care for my two children now that Nyrie would no longer be working for us. Nathaniel would be at school most of the day, but Lucy would only be doing preschool for a few hours three days a week. How on earth would I care for a 4-year-old all day then help my son with his homework and other needs once he got home from school? Paul and I discussed the possibility of putting Lucy into daycare. I didn't want to be separated from my daughter. I wanted to be with her as much as possible, but I knew she would be neglected if she stayed home with me all day. Then, by the time Nathaniel got home from school, I would be so out of my mind with the pain and exhaustion, he would most certainly be neglected as well. I foresaw myself incapacitated, with two children at home, five afternoons a week, and there was no path toward a solution my benzo brain could work out. The guilt I felt over my inability to care for my sweet children made my situation all the more unbearable. I needed help that would allow me to still be a mom, in my own limited way.

That August, before the kids started school, Dan and Delores escaped from the inferno that is Las Vegas during the summer to stay with us as my father-in-law got caught up on the accounting for our business. I watched as my mother-in-law made sure the kids took their nightly baths and read them bedtime stories. I confided in her my misery at the idea of sending Lucy away all day, just because I knew I couldn't make it past lunch without having to lie down for a few hours. "If I could just get some rest, I know I could get through the afternoon until Paul gets home." Paul was in the habit of coming home by 5:30 at the latest to relieve me of my shift, which started when Nyrie left at 4. I could handle more than an hour now that I'd improved a bit with the new medication and daily micro taper. But I couldn't go all day.

"Why don't you ask your neighbors to help?" Delores offered.

"Ask them to watch Lucy every day? That seems like a lot to ask," I despaired.

"It can't hurt to try. You could even offer to pay since you were planning on paying for daycare anyway. Just send out a text and see what happens."

I spent the better part of an hour struggling to combine the phone numbers of moms that I knew with young children in our neighborhood into a group text. I then labored meticulously to craft a brief message. I sent out the text and decided to take a walk around the block to work off the shakiness that followed my exertions. As I walked, I received a reply to my text:

"I can do Wednesdays, no need to pay. My daughters will enjoy having her over to visit."

A second later, I got another response:

"We can do Tuesdays and Thursdays. We love Lucy and could use the extra income."

A few minutes later:

"Mondays work for us, bring her over no charge."

Finally, by the time I got home, I had my last reply:

"I'll take Fridays, no need to pay, we love Lucy."

I couldn't believe it! Within an hour, I had a friend for Lucy to play with every school day of the week in a home with people I knew and trusted. The gratitude I felt was almost as painful as the despair I had felt only a short time earlier at the thought of not being able to care for my daughter. I was overwhelmed. I felt that, maybe, for the first time, God really was watching over my family and me during this ordeal. To this day, I can't express how grateful I am to these women for what they did for my family and me. I didn't have a sufficient explanation at the time as to why I was so incapacitated, and they didn't ask for any justifications from me. They just helped. They may not have known exactly what I was going through, and because of that I don't think they'll ever know how much what they did meant for me, but these women do know what it is to be a mom. They know what it means to serve day and night without any expectation of reward. They know what it is to sacrifice and give and give to those who rarely give back. In other words, they know how to love.

I couldn't repay these moms for what they had done for me. But I could pay it forward.

CHAPTER 12
Transfiguration

Passion is the bridge that takes you from pain to change.

FRIDA KAHLO

Over the next 12 months, I continued my war of attrition with the benzo beast. The monster constantly tried to pull me under the roiling waves as I swam with ever weakening limbs toward a shore I knew must exist ... somewhere. My family, a shimmering mirage on the dark horizon, was my motivation to keep treading water. Help from church members, and the online benzo withdrawal community was my life vest. My neighbor, Lisa, was called to be the relief society president in our ward during that time. I half-jokingly offered her my condolences when I found out. I knew her calling meant hours and hours of time-consuming and emotionally draining volunteer work. I felt the same way when she and several other women during her tenure were assigned to be my visiting teachers. These women were literally required to talk to me and support me spiritually and physically any way they could. I felt bad that all they got from me when they came over was negativity and sadness. Many times I wasn't certain if I would have the strength to entertain the two women who came into my home each month. But it was always worth the effort and the humiliation of failing to look completely sane when they did come over because of what they did for me. It wasn't that they helped me drive my son to school or watch Lucy, although some of them did, it's that they actually listened and seemed to believe me. Despite fruitless efforts to convince doctors and loved ones of the reality and desperate nature of my suffering, I had built in believers at church who regularly came over to listen to me. They sat in my living room, and expressed outrage at the abuses I endured, shed tears for my sorrows, and told me how strong they thought I must be to endure it all. There wasn't much else they could do for me in my condition, but that was all I really needed. They believed me, and that was enough.

I also met online with Jeanette, an energy worker who encouraged me to take the quiet time I had after my mad morning dashes to the toilet, to do a pillar of light meditation, an exercise designed to fill my mind and body with light and energy. She also advised me to do some gentle exercising, read or listen to something spiritual, and keep a gratitude journal. Each morning, before anyone else was up, I would attempt to read a few verses of scripture or listen to talks given by church leaders, then do some light yoga or walking on my air stepper. I don't recall doing the pillar of light exercise faithfully, but I'm sure I tried. As for the journal, I couldn't do much more than scribble out a daily list of things that went right, so that's what I did. At first, it was encouraging, counting my blessings, but after a while, it got depressing. Little changed day after day, whether it was the tasks I could accomplish or the people I encountered. After a few weeks, I began to realize not just how short, but how sadly uniform my lists had become. The following is an example of a particularly eventful day:

June 6

Bathed and fed kids

Took Paul to doctor's

Fed kids lunch

Set up play date for Lucy

Helped Nano play with friend

Helped Paul up the stairs

Made dinner

Read to Lucy

Watched Nano practice piano

Sang to Nano

Helped Lucy get ready for bed

Exercised

Did chakra stones and read a chapter of scripture

Washed towels

Evening nap

Took supplements

Looking at this list, one might think "this was a fairly productive day, not bad." But in looking over it, you have to understand that, anything not written down as one of my daily successes means it didn't happen. For instance, washing the towels was a huge victory, and they most likely also got put in the dryer, but this list says nothing about folding or putting them away. If my daily list doesn't say anything about showering, brushing my hair or getting dressed, then that probably didn't happen either. There's no entry for watching a TV show, talking on the phone with someone, cleaning up the dishes, having a conversation with my husband. Each item I listed took superhuman strength to accomplish. Before attempting many of them, I would have to psych myself up with motivational movie clips like the one from *Lord of the Rings* where Sam carries Frodo up Mount Doom or listen to Rocky's speech to his son in Rocky Balboa. If I didn't have the ability to look up one of these online, I would belt gospel music at the top of my lungs instead: "Just praise through your struggle, and through your pain! Just praise through the storm, yeah through the rain! Beyond every dark cloud, beyond all fear and doubt, there's a blessing, a promise awaiting, in Your praise!"[1] My performances annoyed and often embarrassed my son, particularly whenever he had a friend over to play. But I did what I had to do to survive.

Looking back through my journal of those first few months, I realize that, in some ways, I was a better mother then than I am now. I couldn't do much, but I could sit and hold my children in my arms. I don't do that nearly enough these days. Even though the words stung as a cruel reminder of the joy I used to feel when rocking my babies, I would force the phrase "I love you" out of my mouth as often as I could remember. They were the few words of conversation I could have with my children, and I hoped that they felt something when hearing it, even if my own heart had been turned to lead. Now I can easily feel and express both love and anger, adulation, and annoyance. Sometimes I think I should say less to my children and hold them more.

Three years later, on a rainy November morning, I read the words of my pitifully short list and recognize that today, I am trying to care for my sick son in between Facebooking, writing, reading, fixing my

---

1   Song lyrics from Purple by Donnie McClurkin

hair and makeup, doing my daily load of laundry, and getting in a quick visit to the chiropractor. Maybe later I'll go for a walk if the sun comes out. It's not one of my best days. On those days I'm functioning at about 100 percent. Getting through one of my off days when I have to work with the limitations of my injured brain and body is never easy, but life, for the most part, is really good. I'm even looking forward to watching my weekly show tonight with Paul after the kids are in bed. The sudden realization that almost every single task I fought to accomplish in June of 2014 was entirely for my children explodes in my chest like the gray sheets of rain outside my window. I sob and sob until the storm subsides, and the sun breaks through to illuminate my thoughts. I realize how great my success as a mom was during that horrible time in my life. If it was a choice between doing something for myself or for my family, I chose my family. I made sure that any effort to accomplish anything hour by eternal hour was for my children or my husband in some way, even if they didn't know it. I hoped that subjecting myself to the pain of reading a picture book out loud to Lucy would make up for all the times I couldn't have a conversation with her about her drawings. I hoped that having clean laundry somehow benefitted Nathaniel even though I didn't have the capacity to help him resolve a quarrel or to determine an appropriate response when he felt anxious about going to school. And I hoped with all my heart that on the day Paul had his knee surgery, the day my list was about, he understood how much I sacrificed to help him because that was my only way of showing him I still loved him.

The day of his surgery, after spending grueling hours at the hospital under the bright lights, speaking to strangers, and driving a car, I then had to care for a husband who couldn't climb stairs, when I couldn't even care for myself. I made several trips up and down the stairs to bring him things like food and water. During what I hoped would be my last trip up and down the staircase that night to get Paul ice for his knee, my strength finally gave out. I was too weak even to focus my eyes. I sat at the bottom of the stairs waiting for the courage to make it back up them one more time. Finally, I took a deep breath, turned over onto my hands and knees, and crawled my way up to our bedroom. The effort was so arduous that I had to suck air through my opened mouth as drool dribbled down my chin. Once I got to the top of the stairs, I made one final effort to stand using the wall for support. I tried to put on a brave face for Paul before I entered the bedroom. But he knew I had pushed well past all limits. He volunteered to get his own ice after that, crutches and all.

Difficult as it may be to fathom, that was actually one of my good days, or rather, one of my stronger days. Too many times, I lay in bed, unable to move, listening to my precious children playing outside. Willing my brain and body to get up and check on them, but lacking the mental strength to do it, I would say a silent prayer:

"Please, God, please watch over my children. Please protect them. Make up for my weakness with your grace, through the atonement. You parent them because right now, I cannot."

At other times I lay there lacking the will to hope for anything but an end to my suffering:

Dear Heavenly Father,
I know that if my children were without their mother and my husband without a wife, you would care for them and provide for their needs. You would take care of them for me. Please, if it's your

will, let me die. Give me respite. It's too much to bear. I ran out of strength a long time ago. I won't take my own life. I wouldn't do that to my family. I don't want to hurt them any more than I already have. But if you took me now, there would be no shame or blame. I would be ok with that. I want to feel peace. I want to see Ethan again. Please let me rest.

I heard my answer in the voice of Jean Val Jean speaking to Fantine in *Les Misérables*:

"You have suffered much, poor mother. Oh! do not complain; you now have the dowry of the elect. It is thus that men are transformed into angels."

I would emerge from these deepest, darkest times with a burning passion for saving other souls from falling into this endless pit. I vehemently warned people in support groups who had just cold turkeyed that they only had a short window in which to get back on before the Ashton Manual said it was too late.

"You have no idea, you think you're in cold turkey now, but some people don't experience the full effects of getting off for three or four weeks! It can get so much worse, please, please consider doing a slow taper."

I had been around long enough that I could parrot what I had learned about micro tapering and other advice that was standard in my withdrawal support group. "Wait two to four weeks for your body to adjust after any kind of change in medication or taper protocol."

"A bad wave could be related to so many things. Did your

pharmacy switch brands? Have you introduced any new supplements or changed your diet?"

"You can do this, benzo withdrawal really is that bad, but we really do heal."

I couldn't change what had happened to me. But if I could save just one person from suffering as badly as I was, then my suffering wouldn't be in vain. Toward the end of that year, I was asked if I would assist in the benzo withdrawal support group as a moderator. It was my job to keep track of the conversations, teach newbies the fundamentals, and make sure everyone behaved. Basically, it was like teaching elementary school. Except this online classroom had over 1,000 members, a mere fraction of the membership on BenzoBuddies. I helped people day and night from all over the world, comforting them, defining symptoms, directing them to resources, convincing them to taper more slowly, and generally explaining things in a way that a disoriented, dysfunctional brain could understand.

When I couldn't go downstairs to watch TV with the family because I needed to be in a dark, quiet room (which was always), or when I couldn't have a conversation with my husband because talking made my head vibrate (again, always), I could get online. I could lie on my bed, hold my phone off to the side, squint one eye open to minimize the pain of reading, and help someone through a crisis. Transfigured through the modern miracle of the internet, I was a real person again, a contributing member of society. It was worth it to push through my own emotional pain to help someone else with theirs. When I needed help, I would send voice clips on Facebook Messenger back and forth with my new friends to distract me from what I called the brain pain, the agonizing maddening mental akathisia.

Akathisia is a symptom of an injury usually brought on by neu-rotoxins, such as psychiatric drugs. Someone displaying the physical signs of akathisia looks, well, like a crazy person. They're that person in a mental ward who is rocking back and forth shaking their hands and twitching all over. The movements aren't completely involun-tary. People do it because if they stop, it hurts. The pain of sitting still is worse than the exhaustion of constant motion. When you have akathisia, you can't lie down to sleep, and you can't eat because your fork is moving in as many different directions as your head. One of my friends has had akathisia for years which he developed after tak-ing a prescribed benzodiazepine. He makes YouTube videos about his experience in which you can see how thin he has become from having a body in constant motion. In one of these videos, he comments that akathisia is hell, but that he'd take that any day over the mental akathi-sia he used to get.

Mental akathisia isn't a recognized medical condition, but it's the name we have given to the mental torture many of us benzo warriors experience. Imagine physical akathisia except it's inside your brain. It's mentally painful to sit or lie down. Stilling your mind long enough to focus on a task as simple as writing an email, is agonizing. Your mind is going in a hundred different directions at the same time, and you want it to stop, but all you can do is keep moving, keep distract-ing, keep surviving in the hope that one day, it will end. I'm grateful I never had to deal with physical akathisia, but the mental version was enough to cause me to regularly consider ending my life.

There is no room for God in a brain like that.

My friends in the Christian support groups would often lament that they couldn't feel God anymore. When they would ask me about my beliefs as a "Mormon," I would try my best to answer. Many of my answers sounded surreal in my head. Is this really what I believed? I had no memory of having felt that way about God and the world. Maybe all that was just something that felt familiar or comfortable because I'd grown up with it. I knew my friends were coming to me for spiritual support looking for a reason to keep going, but after a year of heavenly silence, I began to question if there was anyone on the other end of the receiver. Even though I couldn't feel God in my heart or home anymore, I figured, if he was there he probably wasn't ok with me cutting my life short. Besides, I had kids and a husband and people in the support community who looked to me for hope and help. For these reasons, I kept going. I kept acting as if I still believed.

In the meantime, I became friends with a young man who had been involved in a gang shooting. He had been shot in the back and had to go through excruciating therapy to learn how to walk again. The benzodiazepine had been part of his treatment. He told me how getting off of a drug prescribed by his doctor was way worse than any withdrawals he'd experienced from street drugs. He said even getting shot in the back was child's play compared to this new form of torture. Over and over, he would message me, terrified of the constant short-term memory loss he was experiencing, asking if I knew of anyone else as bad as he was. I told him I wasn't sure. I told him that it really was all related to the benzos, that he was young, which increased his chances of healing faster, that yes, I really believed he would get better. Month after month, he would message me, forgetting he had already asked me the exact same questions the other day. Month after month, I would respond, until, one day, he stopped messaging me. His memory returned. He was starting to function normally. I wasn't, but he was, and I was unreservedly happy for him.

I passed on the wisdom handed down to me by my support group mentor: Accept, accept, distract, distract. It's what I did. When my mind was bombarded with looping horrible thoughts that I couldn't control, I found the best distraction was to take those thoughts and turn them into a poem or something funny in my head. Occasionally, I would write them down.

June 23, 2014

10 Reasons Why I Love Recovering From Benzos:

1. My kids' self-esteem has improved now that they're smarter than me.
2. My self-esteem has improved now that I'm smarter than my doctor.
3. All I have to do for Halloween this year is go outside without any makeup on.
4. Memory loss means the same joke can be funny over and over.
5. Memory loss means the same joke can be funny over and over.
6. I've become the world's greatest listener now that I can't think of anything to say.
7. I am no longer at risk for obesity.
8. Nobody can accuse me of sleeping in.
9. I qualify for an Emmy for my efforts at pretending to be normal every day.
10. I have a cool new secret benzo withdrawal code language: ct, dp, sx, wd, lt

My newfound purpose as a support group moderator had its

drawbacks, though. My husband didn't understand why I preferred to be with strangers rather than him, and unless I could type it out, I couldn't reason something like that out well enough to communicate it to him. It's not that I didn't want to be with Paul. I wanted nothing more than for my husband to lie beside me and hold me in the dark. I wanted him to acknowledge the real me that was fighting to communicate with the world outside, and that my way of showing love for him and the kids was by silently suffering rather than drowning them in the tsunami of my pain and fear. But I said none of that. I silently accepted his hurt feelings as a consequence of my condition and beat down the crazy beast that wanted to strike out and hurt him.

Even more frustrating than not being able to make my husband understand, was seeing the same problems over and over again in the online community, and feeling powerless to stop them from happening. People were making themselves worse by going to rehab centers and being treated for addiction when they weren't addicts. Doctors were refusing to help their patients do slow tapers. They were cutting patients off their medication after years, sometimes decades of daily use. How could anyone with any reasonable understanding of how these drugs work believe it was ok to do that to someone? How could they think that a nervous system that has been so drastically altered you could have a seizure and die from suddenly stopping the medication could magically change back to how it used to be in just a few short weeks?

Why weren't these doctors explaining to friends and family that benzodiazepines affect GABA neurons located in 70 percent of cells throughout the brain and body, as well as countless peripheral benzodiazepine receptor cells? Meaning, yes, it can affect their kidneys, or their lungs, or their balance. These receptors do include the immune system, the endocrine system, the skeletal system, and taken altogether, the potential combination of symptoms is practically infinite! This means that no, your loved one isn't making this all up, they really are sick, and they need your help. Why didn't the people I was helping have access to knowledgeable doctors or even a legitimate diagnosis so they could apply for disability? Why didn't the drug companies provide us with medications that could be safely tapered so we didn't have to create drug labs in our kitchens and bathrooms in order to wean off slow enough to avoid a stroke or seizure? Why were women, disabled by withdrawal, left with no other option but to give up their children to abusive ex-spouses? Why were chemists, teachers, and nurses reduced to homelessness? Where was the outrage, the news stories, the call for legislative action?

I had to do something.

In the spring of 2015, almost exactly a year after beginning my taper, I made my own YouTube video. Actually, I begged Paul to help me make it since I didn't know how. I had to convince him to do it. He was worried that putting myself out there online like that might expose me, and our family to all the potential nut jobs on the internet. But I felt compelled to do it, and he knew I would go even crazier than I already was if I didn't. One evening, while I was in the middle of a particularly good window, I offered a quick prayer asking God to help me say the words that needed saying. Then I sat in front of the computer in Paul's office and made the kind of video that I would want to show to others, a video that explained what this illness was in a compassionate, relatable way. I didn't want anybody I knew in real life to see it. I didn't like the idea of friends or acquaintances watching me bare my soul on camera. I hoped they wouldn't. I did it for the people I was trying to help online. I knew how hard it was to try and explain what was going on inside your body to others when you didn't fully understand it yourself. So I made a video that said it for them. Before I published it, I said another prayer. "Heavenly Father, please, I want to help as many people as I can. Please help as many people as possible to see this. But if you do, then please protect me. I can't do this if I have to face negativity and online bullying. I can't handle anything like that right now. If you want me to do this, then I need your protection. Please, bless my work." And he did.

I never planned on having a YouTube channel with thousands of followers. I just had something that needed to be said and felt compelled to say it. I made another impromptu video just a week and a half later, during a rather extraordinary window of clarity during a bout of stomach flu. It was after yet another abusive interview with a doctor for my prescription refill. I was angry and needed to speak out. My video, entitled "Benzo Bullied, you're not crazy!" was picked up by Mad in America, an online webzine focused on the abuses of psychiatry and education towards reform. When I made my first video, I thought it would be cool if one day it got a thousand views. My Benzo Bullied video got more than that in a few days. After that, I decided to do more than just talk. I wanted to provide education for patients, doctors, and friends and family of benzo victims, that was compelling and backed by scientific literature. My next videos were about tapering strategies and the science behind benzodiazepine withdrawal syndrome. The latter had pop-ups with references to all the research supporting my statements. All of a sudden, I was getting tens of thousands of views on videos about a dry, obscure subject that, while lacking any entertainment value, was also somewhat controversial. During all that time, I never had one negative comment on any of my videos, even though professional online trolls regularly stalked the benzo community. The only explanation I could come up with for the success of my videos was God and that more people than I could have realized desperately needed the hope and information I was providing.

And still, it wasn't enough.

We were getting floods of new people into the online support community every day, and things only seemed to be getting worse. Doctors were ripping patients off their benzodiazepines because they were getting in trouble for overprescribing. Patients were dismissed as addicts or noncompliant, even when they were tapering off their benzos. The misprescribing, misdiagnosing, unnecessary surgeries and medications, all of it was getting worse.

One of my friends asked me to help her run an online group focused on gathering members and data for a class action lawsuit. I hate litigation. It was one of the most stressful things I ever had to deal with when I was well and able, but now, I couldn't imagine how upsetting it would be. But then, I also couldn't ignore the cries for justice and change. I finally acquiesced when I realized that the group we would form could focus on so much more. Benzo warriors needed a place to discuss the role of the media and legislation in this problem. They needed help applying for disability and finding lawyers who would help them file medical malpractice claims. People in our community needed a place where they felt empowered to speak out about this problem without being overwhelmed by the daily accounts of personal tragedy. This was no support group. It was a battlefield.

Our phones and laptops became our greatest weapons as we

jumped into the hairy crossfires of online activism. We initiated letter-writing campaigns to editors of newspapers who completely misrepresented the benzo problem and misinformed the public with dubious facts and opinions. We sought out the doctors quoted in these articles who said things like, "benzos are safer than aspirin," and bombarded them with emails. Even when writing a few paragraphs was physically painful for our members, they did it anyway, because it gave a purpose to their suffering. Many of these people were so brain damaged, myself included, that we spent a good portion of our time guiding them through the process of sending a simple email or downloading and uploading files. But that's the miracle of social media. Even a weak and humble minority can fight back.

People from outside the support community began reaching out to us. An award-winning film director needed people to interview for a documentary she was making about benzo syndrome. I was asked to be one of the subjects in her movie. Paul and I prayed about it and decided this would be one of the best opportunities we would have to really make a difference. We agreed to have a film crew come to our home and document our lives.

But it still wasn't enough.

The movie would be years in the making. Meanwhile, the legal action group wasn't powerful enough to influence the day to day prescribing of doctors, the main front on which this battle was being fought. A lawsuit was becoming less and less likely as none of the numerous law firms we reached out to would consider taking the case. We got close once, but they became skittish when they realized how powerful the pharmaceutical industry's influence really was. Big Pharma had way too many laws protecting it, not surprising given they spend more on lobbying than big tobacco, big oil, and big defense combined. This war would have to be won in the court of public opinion. We needed a more authoritative voice speaking to doctors, legislators, and the media. I asked my partner in the legal action group if she would take the next step with me and start a nonprofit. Now it was her turn to be reluctant. It took a couple of months of my friend experiencing the same frustrating impotence I had been subjected to through my work as a support group moderator and on my channel before she finally changed her mind.

After countless hours spent creating content for the website and our new YouTube channel, we officially launched the Benzodiazepine Information Coalition (BIC) nonprofit. God had been good; I could see his hand in its creation. He had orchestrated many things, opened windows, inspired hearts. Of course, he had. Our Father in heaven wanted to help his children as much as I did. Why wouldn't he want to right this wrong? Finally! Benzo sufferers would have a voice that could be heard in the media, in doctors' offices, and be taken seriously by loved ones looking for an authority on the subject. Finally, I would have the power to really help people. I had recently finished my taper and was starting to see some improvements. I had so many ideas and dreams, yes, dreams. They could really be a part of my life again. I had done so much research and witnessed countless case studies over the past year and a half. I had basically earned my master's in benzodiazepines. Was there a degree for that? I could see the day when I might be well enough to go back to school and further my education in a way that would benefit my work with BIC. I had plans.

God's were just a little different than mine.

CHAPTER 13

Physician Heal Thyself

If you are deemed insane, then all actions that would otherwise prove you are not, do, in actuality, fall into the framework of an insane person's actions. Your sound protests constitute denial. Your valid fears are deemed paranoia. Your survival instincts are labeled defense mechanisms. It's a no-win situation. It's a death penalty really.

DENNIS LEHANE, SHUTTER ISLAND

"People are told all the time that their mental illness is like diabetes. 'You wouldn't expect a person with diabetes to just stop taking their insulin, would you? It's the same with your depression or your anxiety. You need this to correct the imbalance in your brain.'"

I repeated these words as I sat across the table from Dr. Wright, an addiction and pain management specialist I had met seven months earlier at the 2017 International Benzodiazepine Symposium in Bend, Oregon. I had been included as part of a panel discussion on the effects of long-term benzodiazepine use. We had kept in touch since the symposium and, as he had a speaking engagement in Utah that week, Dr. Wright had invited my husband and me to meet him for breakfast that morning in Salt Lake.

"I've never heard that; that's not what we tell our patients," the good doctor replied.

"Trust me," I said, "people are told this all the time. It's how doctors get their patients to be compliant when they start questioning whether the drugs they're taking are hurting more than they're helping."

I liked talking with Dr. Wright; he was always up for a good debate. He welcomed everyone to the International Benzodiazepine Symposium on the first day by opening his presentation with "Hello, I'm Doctor Wright, and I'm a recovering benzodiazepine prescriber." He, like so many other practitioners who attended the symposium last fall had been converted by the testimonies of patients like myself who spoke to the horrors of benzodiazepine syndrome. But like many who sympathize with our plight, he still believed antidepressants and drugs like gabapentin were good, safe alternatives. My experience in helping hundreds of benzo victims from all over the world who were also on multiple psychiatric medications led me to believe otherwise. Antidepressants, anticonvulsants, antipsychotics, all of them could be just as harmful.

It was incredible that I was sitting here calmly having this discussion with a doctor even as I was dealing with some of the lingering effects of my brain/body injury. My past experiences with the medical profession had not been so positive. From the day I was born I had been violated by doctors. The scars on either side of my face are from the OB/GYN who was in a hurry to deliver me because he had a golf tournament to attend. Rather than wait for my mother to push through the rest of an already rapid labor, he grabbed the forceps and yanked me out so hard, it sliced my face, just above the inside of my ear lobes. But this is insignificant to what was to come in the years following.

The irony in tapering off a benzodiazepine is that you have to keep taking it. Week after week, month after month, I reduced my prescription by such minute amounts (roughly 0.05 mg) that, by medical standards, it was insignificant. Every morning, I made up my liquid suspension by dropping the Valium pills in 300 ml of water then shaking that up and removing 1 ml more than the day before with a syringe. Twice a day I recoiled from the poison I was forced to drink. I saw myself as Dumbledore in the cave by the sea with Harry Potter, willingly drinking the potion of despair, yet crying, pleading, raging at being made to so. They say the only way out of hell is to keep going. For me, it was to keep drinking. Sip by sip; I drained the waters of the lake of fire and brimstone. Milliliter by milliliter, I got closer and closer to freedom.

Of course, in order to do this, I had to get refills of my prescription. This meant walking into the lion's den once a month, sitting there with the electronic sign-in pad on my lap, debating whether or not to document which symptoms I was currently experiencing. Clicking on every one of the 30 or so symptoms I had on any given day was not only a waste of time, but it also subjected me to the irony of ironies, an advertisement for the pills their algorithm determined was best suited to treat my condition, the panacea miracle cure, psychiatric drugs.

"You're too pretty to scar," was Dr. Scott's way of trying to convince me to treat the boils that began to erupt, with Accutane or some type of antibiotic. The one comfort I'd had throughout my hellish withdrawal was that my skin was clear. I didn't have the energy to fix my hair or put on makeup, but I could wear a hat and look ok. In fact, I was down to my pre-pregnancy, pre-Cymbalta weight, and fitting into clothes that I hadn't worn in years. At least I could sort of look normal even if I couldn't act normal. Then, like Job, that too was taken from me and I was cursed with boils. I didn't know what they were at first. The red hot eruptions would get so large, one I had on my eyebrow obstructed my vision, another under my lower lip made it hard for me to close my mouth, causing me to drool. I thought it was really bad cystic acne. The first dermatologist Paul took me to didn't even question my self-diagnosis. I could tell he was in a hurry. He pulled out his scalpel, sliced open my "cysts" and dug around to "break them up." I went home and applied wet heat to help them drain as he had instructed. That visit took a lot out of me. When my skin started sagging in the places he had cut, like it was melting off my face, I didn't have the energy to care. I didn't have the wherewithal to call, set up a follow-up appointment, get Paul to drive me back to his office, and confront him. I just lived with it. I still live with it today, with scars so severe I look like I was both in a knife fight and have some really weird, misplaced dimples.

"I can prescribe an antibiotic or some Accutane. You're too pretty to scar." He repeated at each visit.

"I can't, I'm too sensitive," was the extent of my counter-argument.

The last antibiotic I took during withdrawal made me suicidal. As for Accutane, a drug with that many side effects that can cause depression? No way. I had already gone crazy on the Prozac I was prescribed by a supposed withdrawal expert down in Provo. I had made the 20-minute drive south to see him sometime towards the beginning of my taper in 2014. I was desperate to find anyone who could help me develop an Ashton taper program. This doctor came recommended by a family member back east who also practiced medicine.

Nice looking and younger than expected, he sat across from me on his swivel stool.

"Have you ever heard of the Ashton Manual?" I inquired. "It says to do a slow taper and do a crossover to Valium. Do you understand how to do a crossover? I just switched in one day, and I'm wondering if that's part of my problem."

"I've helped lots of patients get off benzos," the doctor replied. "You're overthinking things, just cut your dose by 2 or 3 mg this week, and I'll prescribe you some Prozac to help with the symptoms."

He got out his prescription pad. "Prozac is like the red-headed stepchild of antidepressants these days," he joked, "but it's actually still one of the best treatment options."

I tried to explain to him that this wasn't your typical case of withdrawal. I tried to tell him this went way beyond depression. I had already taken Cymbalta. It didn't seem like a good idea to me now to take Prozac. I don't know if I just didn't do a good job of explaining or he just didn't do a good job of listening, but with a sympathetic tone in his voice, he bulldozed through my concerns. "Life is hard. It's hard being a stay at home mom, all day every day. Some people just can't handle being moms. My wife is that way. It's just too hard for her, and she needs some help." With the understanding that "help" meant meds, he handed me the prescription for Prozac. I walked down the stairs to my car, thinking maybe he was right. The last time I was bad like this I'd just had Lucy. Maybe I wasn't as strong as I thought I was. Maybe I just couldn't handle being a mom.

Three days later, I lie in my bed unable to move or speak. I had spent the previous two days manic, unable to stop going, going despite the pain and fatigue. I simply couldn't stop! When I called the doctor, I told him that I read something on the NIH, which says not to prescribe a full dose of Prozac to someone with any sort of severe anxiety condition. He told me to cut my dose in half, much good that did. What little energy I had to exist from day to day had been spent. My friends in the support group had told me not to take any antidepressants, but I didn't listen. I wanted to try at least. I wanted to believe that somebody out there with a medical degree knew how to help me. But it was becoming increasingly apparent none of them understood or believed what I had to say. And really, how can you help someone you don't even believe?

From then on, I decided that doctors served only one purpose, to refill my prescription. The only people who had ever truly helped me were those in the support group. The only doctor I trusted was Heather Ashton, and she lived on the other side of the Atlantic. I was on my own. I had a doctor who was willing to prescribe Valium, and that was more than many in the benzo community had.

The only time I ever felt like Dr. Scott truly believed me, was in December of 2014 when, once again, he urged me to take something to treat the boils that continued to disfigure my face.

"There has to be a reason why this is happening." He anxiously implored, "Are your periods still regular?"

"Yes."

"Have you started taking anything different?"

"No."

"Are you eating differently? Maybe it's an allergy."

"I eat clean as I always have, no wheat, no dairy, no processed foods."

"Is there anything you can think of that has changed?"

"The only thing that's changed is that I've been withdrawing from Valium," I stated with finality.

Dr. Scott paused. A moment of silence passed before he responded.

"Then maybe you should hold off on tapering for a while. Just stay where you are and give your body a chance to calm down. See if that helps."

It actually did help. But I couldn't stay at 7 mg forever. Besides, Dr. Scott's position was becoming precarious. He'd been flagged by the DEA for his prescribing of controlled substances. Mid-taper, I was made to sign a contract stating I was not doctor or pharmacy shopping, or abusing my prescription. I also had to agree to give urine samples. I found it ironic that the very year I was actually trying to stop taking a controlled substance, I was being treated like a junkie. I prayed every time I entered his office, that this would not be the month he decided to cut me off from my prescription, as I had seen happen to so many others in the support groups. Doctors were getting jumpy as they saw other prescribers getting into trouble, and their patients were paying the price. I was lucky to have a doctor with whom I had a rapport, who knew me before the benzos.

The only problem was that he was always out of town.

Several times throughout my 15-month long taper with Valium, I had to see another doctor at Premier Family Medical to get my prescription refilled. Twice I had to schedule a visit with Dr. Keith, once in 2014 and once in 2015. He was a respected physician and member of the local legislature. That first visit, he asked me many questions about my taper. Why was I going so slow? Why was I using 10 and 2 mg pills? Why couldn't I just take an antidepressant instead? He asked if I had a family history of mental illness. "No." Addiction? "No." I told him, "I tried getting off faster. I tried an antidepressant. Believe me, I want nothing more than to be off this stuff. But even though tapering is making me sick, I was much worse before. I would do anything, anything to avoid going through that again." I explained how I learned to taper from the Ashton Manual, how this had saved my life. He didn't care.

"Well, if I were your doctor, I wouldn't touch this taper plan with a ten-foot pole," was Dr. Keith's response.

I was shaking. I struggled every second I sat there, just to keep breathing and not black out. It took every ounce of strength I had to explain my situation to him, yet somehow he was entitled to simply dismiss everything I had just said? I didn't want to argue. I was terrified he wouldn't refill my prescription and then where would I be?

"Well, if you have a better solution, I'm open to hearing it." I politely responded, "I certainly don't enjoy month after month of withdrawal."

"That's what pain clinics and detox centers are for," he spat back.

"I already called a detox center. They said they couldn't help me, that I was already getting myself off and they had nothing to offer me."

That shut him up ... until the next time I had to get my refill.

This time I tried to make myself look more presentable. I spent the morning covering my boils with half an inch of makeup. It was a struggle as the image in the mirror was blurry. Raising my arms above my head to style my hair was like trying to carry a bag of cement uphill while holding my breath. Sweating from the exertion of energy I did not have; I was determined to make myself not look like a junkie or a mental case.

That wintry afternoon I sat in the same chair in the same room of the upper floor office at Premier. My head swimming, I calmly and respectfully responded to every question Dr. Keith shot at me. In the back of my mind I thought, "Wow, he's really intent on hearing what I have to say! Maybe something I said last time sparked something in him, and he really wants to understand." As I finished up my summary of the Ashton Manual and how it has helped countless members of the support community get successfully and permanently off their benzos he interjected,

"That's all pseudoscience."

WHAT? He made me go through all that just so he could make that statement?! I don't remember how I responded, but Dr. Keith's next comment was:

"Well, if you're so smart then what do you need us dumb doctors for?"

Surprised by the increased hostility in his countenance, I opened my mouth, then closed it. Then with a flat stare, I spoke the last two words I would ever have to say to Dr. Keith,

"For refills."

To my surprise, I walked out of Premier that day with my prescription for Valium.

A mere two years later, I sat across from an addiction specialist who respectfully listened as he and I debated whether various psychiatric medications were reasonable treatments for someone with a benzodiazepine injury.

"You have to be very careful," Dr. Wright said with concern, "You don't want to be held liable for practicing medicine without a license."

He wasn't necessarily referring to my channel, but to the many people who had reached out to me, offering to pay for my services if I would help them develop a withdrawal schedule and counsel them through their tapers.

"I know," I said, "I get that, but what can we do to help these people? Their doctors don't know how to help them, and they need professional help. People are dying because their doctors refuse to read the Ashton Manual even when it's placed right in their laps! Our biggest problem right now is that we can't get doctors to prescribe to people who WANT to get off their benzos. They're perfectly willing to prescribe for years and years, but as soon as someone is ready to withdraw, they say, 'ok, I'm giving you four weeks to get off and then that's it, no more refills after that.' Look at the comments under my videos. People are suffering. I know what they're going through and I can't just sit back and do nothing."

I felt impotent. Like many benzo warriors before me, I poured my heart and soul into creating the kind of change that might save others from this awful fate. Benzo warriors managed all the current websites and support groups. I co-founded the Benzodiazepine Information Coalition along with two other leaders in the support community. It was a benzo survivor who organized and funded the International Benzodiazepine Symposium. Most recently, a businessman, the husband of a nurse who had been disabled by benzo withdrawal syndrome, spearheaded an alliance of doctors and researchers from the symposium who were determined to research this illness and educate their peers. And yet none of that seemed to make a difference when someone came to me desperate for the kind of help only a doctor was legally permitted to provide. But now, doctors were finally taking on the responsibility so many of us had shouldered for decades. Maybe it was time for the sick and the disabled to step back and let the people who should have been helping us all along, take up the banner and run, where we could only crawl.

Dr. Wright brought up the idea of creating a new benzo withdrawal workbook and manual as part of his efforts at the Alliance for Benzodiazepine Best Practices, the nonprofit which emerged from the International Benzodiazepine Symposium. I had been brought on as an advisor at the request of some of its members. He would write the technical manual geared towards medical professionals, and I would co-author the workbook for patients. I'd had many people request the exact same thing from me on my channel. The Ashton Manual was great, but a workbook and updated manual was the next logical step. Everything was falling into place.

I had to leave the Benzodiazepine Information Coalition soon after its inception and it broke my heart. I'd failed to finish the work I had set out to accomplish. I prayed it would continue to do some good. But my failures with BIC fortuitously led to my involvement with the Alliance. Now there were two nonprofits. It seemed like God was orchestrating something grander for those who were suffering than what I had originally intended, and I was content to be his instrument.

CHAPTER 14

True Love

All, everything that I understand, I understand only because I love.

LEO TOLSTOY, WAR AND PEACE

Holly's crew finished arranging the cameras and lights on Paul who was sitting on a barstool in the middle of our entryway from the living room to the kitchen. I had already been interviewed earlier that day for the *As Prescribed* film about my benzodiazepine injury. The filtered lights cast a halo around Paul in the center of our home. The neighbors were helping us watch the kids so we could focus on the interview. I didn't want to go upstairs and lie all alone in my bed while everyone was downstairs, so I opted for the couch.

It had been a rough day. The anticipation of the film crew arriving at our home had made it difficult for me to get much sleep the night before. It had only been a couple of months since I finished my taper and while I had improved some, I was still pretty disabled, especially on days like today. Plus, talking all day to people while trying to put on a brave face was grueling. I was shaking. I had to keep taking breaks throughout my interview to walk off the nervous energy or lie down to try and breathe through the disorientation that was still my constant companion.

Now it was Paul's turn. I wanted to watch him, but it was too painful to focus my eyes, so I just lay there and breathed, in and out, listening as he and the director, Holly Hardman, chatted about what to expect during the interview. Then they started recording. I heard Paul talk about what it was like to be a loved one taking care of a benzo victim. I was familiar with his struggle, taking over the role I used to play in our family, advocating for me with friends and relatives, his feelings of helplessness as he watched me suffer. I knew it wasn't easy for him to talk about all that, but I was glad he had the opportunity to get it all out there, to be validated by this experience. Being in a film about people like us made his story important, it lent meaning to this tragedy.

As Paul shared his thoughts on how I had improved over the last few months, Holly asked him, "When did you know Jocelyn would get better?" Paul answered, "I didn't." His answer hit me square in the face. Stunned by the blow, I quickly turned the other cheek and listened this time with both ears. "I wasn't sure if she would ever get better." What?! I silently shouted, staring daggers at him from behind closed eyes. I had always thought Paul believed, as I did, the accounts of all the people who had healed from this illness. Their stories gave me a hope to which I had clung for the past year and a half. How could he have gotten through all this without that belief? Was it his experience with his dad's brain injury that gave him the fortitude to stick it out with me? Suddenly, it made sense why night after night, I would ask Paul if he thought I would get better, and night after night, he would never give me a direct answer. I believed I would. I hoped I would, but I asked him because I needed to hear it from his lips. I needed the reassurance that someone else believed it too. For all the countless ways in which Paul was there for me, he never could bring himself to tell me I would get better. Now I finally understood why. It hurt to know that the whole time I was giving hope to others through my videos and in the support groups, the one person I had failed to convince was my husband. Paul kept talking to Holly.

"I thought she might be that way for the rest of our lives and so I started to make plans for caring for her in the future."

I listened bitterly as Paul went into the details of how he planned to care for his disabled wife over the next few decades. I was so grateful to him for everything he had done and was still doing for our family. I didn't want to be angry with Paul for lacking faith in me. I sifted through the darkness of my muddled brain for a better way to look at this. Then, in that singular moment, my mind was illuminated by the realization that Paul was planning on staying with me for the rest of my life, no matter what! Even though I was no longer a partner in our relationship or contributing in any substantial way, even though I was no longer talented, or beautiful, or witty, or fun, he was planning on being with me and caring for me throughout our marriage. Not just until death do us part, but for eternity as he had promised to do when he knelt across from me on the altar in the Salt Lake Temple. I shrank from the belief that this could be possible. Why would he do that? Why would he even consider being with me for the rest of my miserable life when his held so much promise?

Then the answer filled my soul. Because he loves me. He loved me even when boils covered my face, and my hair was falling out. He loved me when I couldn't read our children a bedtime story or crack jokes at the dinner table. His love wasn't based on how talented I was or how much I could contribute financially. He simply loved me, and that meant I was worthy of love even when I had nothing of worth to offer.

I used to feel a sense of worth from knowing that I had a Father in Heaven who loved me. I hadn't always had this gift. It started when I was 13 years old and feeling worthless. I was miserable at home, I didn't feel like I had any friends at school, and I hated life. I would make excuses or pretend to be sick, so I didn't have to go to Pitts, the ironic name of my middle school. One evening, I attended a youth fireside that was a part of our church youth conference. One of the speakers talked about his determination in high school to read the scriptures for an hour every day. He would get up at 5:30 a.m. just so he could read his scriptures before attending early morning seminary on weekdays before school. After the fireside, the rest of the kids all went off to get ready for the dance that would be starting in another hour. At thirteen, I wouldn't be old enough to attend the dance until the next year, so I went out into the foyer of our stake building to wait for my ride with the rest of the 12- and 13-year-olds.

One by one, they all got into their cars and rode away until I was left alone. As I sat by myself on that orange polyester couch, separated by a glass partition from the rest of the building, I began to cry for no particular reason. I never cried in those days and certainly never in public. But I couldn't help myself, and I continued to cry for what must have been 20 minutes at least. By that time the speaker had finally extricated himself from all the people who'd come up to chat with him and shake his hand after the fireside. He was walking out to his car when he came across me silently sobbing in the dark. He sat down next to me and asked me what was wrong. I told him I didn't know. I was never very good at delving into feelings. He tried to probe some more, but I was a brick wall. He asked if he could do anything for me, and I said no. Then he asked if he could make a request of me. I gave my assent. He asked me if I would promise him to start reading the scriptures every day. I considered what he said and realized it was the answer to the question I never thought to ask, the question that had been dissolving my stony heart to tears ... 'What's wrong with my life?' I knew I needed to change something, and as soon as he said it, I knew this was the way. The room suddenly grew brighter, and I felt a sense of hope enter my soul. Yes, I would read the scriptures every day, starting with the Book of Mormon. In fact, I silently told myself I would read them every day for an hour just as he had done. That was the summer before 7th grade.

Every night after dinner, I would go to my bedroom, open up my Book of Mormon, and read for an hour. Eventually, it turned into half an hour and then 15 to 20 minutes. But without fail, every single night, I would read my scriptures no matter what. Things started to change. Not that my life circumstances changed in any way. Those remained the same. But *I* changed. I began to feel like I was special, like I had someone who knew me and was aware of me all the time. I felt loved. I had the desire to share that love with others. Life became something worth living.

But benzos had taken that from me. I couldn't feel God's love, no matter how much I prayed or how much I listened to the scriptures when I couldn't read them, it was like he had disappeared. My source of love and worth was gone. One by one, all the measurable things that made me feel like a valuable human being had been stripped from me until nothing but an empty carcass remained. If there was a God, then he had left me to rot. I loathed the stench of my cadaverous remains.

But then I heard Paul reveal his love for me when I was at my very worst. In an instant, the dawn of love pierced my pain, breaking through the darkness in my soul and I was reborn. I remembered what it felt like to be truly loved. I realized that my whole life, there had always been a part of me that believed I had to earn love in some way, whether through obedience and goodness, excelling in my studies or looking perfect. I never accepted another human being could love me just because I was me. This belief meant there was always a part of myself that I held back from my husband. I never completely trusted him. If he was going to hurt me, I wanted to be able to shut myself off from him as easily as I had from the other painful things in my life. And he had hurt me, many times. Only the people we truly care about can hurt us as they do. Still, as I lay on that couch in the darkness, much like the one I sat on 24 years ago, I learned the meaning of true love.

I trusted in my husband's love for me and anchored myself to the belief that it was a representation of the love of God I had so desperately been seeking. From then on, even with all the trauma and confusion and pain, my relationship with my husband blossomed in a way it never had before.

CHAPTER 15

Date Nights

The wound is the place where the Light enters you.

Paul and I continued our weekly tradition of Friday date nights that started, ironically enough, the weekend before my miscarriage two years earlier.

We had asked my parents to watch the kids for us while we went to the ER. After they found out I might be having a miscarriage they offered to take the kids for the entire weekend. Yes, the news of the miscarriage was upsetting, especially after already losing one baby and almost losing the second, but it paled in comparison to everything else I was going through. This wasn't the time to mourn over the future. The present loomed monstrously vast, making it impossible to envision anything else. The doctor had given me diazepam, and I was feeling kind of stable for the first time in months. I still couldn't do much, but there was one thing I could do. I could accept Paul's offer to go out to dinner with him that evening. I knew how much he needed to break up the monotony of the past two months he'd spent caring day and night for an invalid while parenting two little children. I didn't want to do it, but I did it for him.

We weren't in the habit of going out to eat, but when we did, Paul and I were used to eating cheap, which meant fast food. Of course, now I was never hungry, and as for taste, if it didn't taste like metal, then food didn't taste like anything at all. Paul decided Panda Express sounded good and I had no reason to argue with that. When we pulled up to the restaurant, I told Paul I couldn't face all those people inside. I didn't know why. I'd never had agoraphobia before, so I didn't have a name for my problem. I just knew that it was too much to bear. I hid my face from the worker at the drive-through by pretending to look out the passenger window while resting my head on my left hand. Paul gave her our order then drove to a spot in the parking lot that faced away from the restaurant. My husband and I sat in that parked car in silence as we ate our orange chicken and walnut shrimp. It was the first night of our new weekly ritual. From then on, Paul insisted on our getting out of the house once a week, every Friday when he got home from work, no matter how bad things got. There were still many Friday evenings when I was too sick to even get up from my bed. But if I could put one foot in front of the other, no matter how much mental or physical pain I was in, we went on a date.

I would bear the car ride in silence to whichever destination my husband chose, then bury my face in his arm as he walked me to the back of whichever restaurant we entered. I can't say I enjoyed our date nights. Fun and other such pleasant feelings were no longer a part of my emotional vocabulary. Heaven knows it was incredibly difficult for me to engage the fine motor skills and visual acuity it took to put on makeup and fix my hair, the results of which were mostly abysmal. But I did it anyway, because I knew he needed it, and because it broke up the monotony of suffering alone in my room all day. I did it because it meant I didn't have to worry for a few hours about failing to be the mother my children needed me to be every single minute of every day. I did it because; what else was I going to do?

We started eating at much nicer restaurants because they weren't as bright and noisy as fast food joints. Paul would ask to be seated in a dark corner somewhere, so I would have to make as little eye contact with people as possible. I made sure to keep my head down as he ordered the food for me. I was never able to finish a meal. The sensation of being full would only serve to aggravate my symptoms even more. I nibbled. I attempted to talk with my husband a little. But mostly I would look at my phone for distraction, reading the posts of other benzo sufferers online. After dinner, Paul and I would splurge on a movie. The kind you go to see in an actual auditorium, not the ones you pick up from a red box outside of Walgreens. Whereas before, our occasional date nights involved free activities like browsing through bookstores or museums, now we had to do something that required as little effort as possible. A dark movie theater seemed like the best option.

I recall waiting with bated breath until the theater lights dimmed, and I could finally be bathed in darkness. Exposing my heightened senses to the flashing images on the screen and the booming bass of surround sound was excruciating, but at least no one was looking at me. For some reason, I never thought to bring earplugs (until someone from a benzo support group mentioned it). I would watch the screen with one eye open, then switch to the other eye, tilting my head likewise. I spent much of those movies leaning forward with my head buried in my hands. When the back pain got too bad, I would push past my fear of being noticed by other people to stand and walk to the back of the theater where I could shift from one foot to the other, or lean over an empty chair to ease the shooting pains in my back and neck.

One night, Paul took me to see *Unbroken*, the story of WWII hero Louis ("Louie") Zamperini. I couldn't handle action films or horror movies anymore (my life had become a horror story, I certainly didn't need to see that played out on a big screen) and while this movie was neither of those, it was still overwhelming. But something about this man's suffering broke through my wall of pain and pricked at the emotions buried under its rubble. Louie was a WWII pilot who got stranded on a life raft in the middle of the Pacific Ocean for 47 days. Picked up by the Japanese, he spent the rest of the war in a prisoner-of-war camp. He endured torture at the hands of a merciless villain. I could relate to that, and I wanted to know more.

When my neighbor, Lisa, came to visit me soon after, I discovered she had a copy of the book *Unbroken*. Even though I couldn't read very well, I asked to borrow it. I read in five-to-ten-minute increments, one eye closed, switching from my left eye to the right. Sometimes I would lie on my back, head hanging over the edge of the bed and read upside down. I did whatever it took to unearth the hope I felt must lay hidden somewhere within those pages. When Delores visited, I asked her if she could read a bit of my book to me, after all, she read to the kids every night, but she declined. I asked my husband; I even asked my 8-year-old son, who was an avid reader, to read some of it to me. It broke my heart that no one did. Nevertheless, I felt compelled to finish the story, and so, battling through the brain pain, I read on.

I found out Louie had been experimented on, injected with a poison that could have killed him. I could relate to that; even though a doctor had prescribed my poison, it was no less toxic to my body. I felt Louie's hunger as I read about him being starved by the prison guards. Nobody was forcibly withholding food from me. My prison guard was my own fear and pain. Terrified that putting the wrong substance in my mouth would bring on vertigo, akathisia or worsen the neuralgia as it had in the past, I would stand in front of the fridge for ten or fifteen minutes several times a day, trying to discern which foods were "safe" to eat. Inevitably, I would simply give up and walk away. Any sustenance I did receive was denied by my body anyway. The food that entered my stomach went straight through my bowels and into the toilet. As I walked the border of the neighborhood that was my prison camp, pondering the most recent chapter of *Unbroken*, I came across Lisa tending to her garden. Despite my attempt at avoiding eye contact, she observed the loose clothes hanging off my atrophied figure and cried out, "Oh my gosh! You've lost MORE weight?" a look of concern on her face. "Yeah, haha. That's the benefit of not being able to eat anything," I joked and walked on. The irony of my prison was that I was the only one who could see the bars.

I didn't need a sadistic figure shouting abusive language at me night and day. My own brain managed that very well. And as for the beatings Louie received, well, I always felt like I had just woken up the day after a beating. Sometimes I would lose the ability to use a limb, or my muscles would seize so severely that my own spasming would pop a shoulder or rib so out of joint that it hurt just to breathe. Other times I would get a sharp, stabbing pain on the side of my face as though someone had stuck a hot needle in my eardrum. I could go on and on with the physical torture I endured, but none of that compared to the rape of my mind and body that was benzodiazepine withdrawal syndrome. I was violated night and day by an invisible entity and to make things worse; there was no one to accuse, no one I could point the finger at and say, "You are my enemy!" Stories like Louie's and those of concentration camp victims were the only examples extreme enough for me to relate to, not just because they suffered so much, but because they endured all that and made it out alive. Even more hopeful to me was the knowledge that many of them, like Louie Zamperini, went on to live good lives.

As I read past the part where Louie's story in the movie ended, I found out he returned home with severe PTSD. Louie had nightmares about his prison guards every night, which left him sleep-deprived and traumatized. I, on the other hand, had something known as rebound dreaming. When you don't dream for years, it's like your body is trying to make up for all that lost REM sleep. That's when the rebound dreaming kicks in. I would have what felt like hour after hour of vivid, violent, and terrifying dreams. Although I prayed day and night for relief from the exhaustion and to escape the hell of wakefulness, rebound dreaming made sleep deprivation preferable to what happened when I was unconscious. Upon waking after a fitful night's sleep or an afternoon nap, I would find myself more exhausted and frightened by the dreams I'd had than when I went to bed. And then there was toxic sleep. Something about the sleep process caused my body to detox. I would wake up feeling as though I had been poisoned, cramping, debilitated by the pain in my face and neck, and completely unable to focus my eyes. This combined with the horrifying images that played out in my mind night after night left me feeling traumatized and violated, as though my mind had been raped every night that I went to sleep. I feared going to bed. But I feared being awake too.

It might be surprising to hear that, for me, being up all night wasn't all bad. Often, I found a sense of peace somewhere in the middle of the night when everyone was asleep. It's like a switch flipped on in my brain, and I was normal for an hour or two. On warm summer nights, I would take a walk around the neighborhood at 2 or 3 o'clock in the morning, drinking in the quiet darkness that enveloped me. That was the good part. The bad part was what I called the "witching hour" that usually followed. These were the early hours of the morning after a sleepless night, around 4 or 5 a.m. when the prospect of facing a new day loomed on the horizon. This is when I felt the terror rise in my throat. I couldn't rationalize it away. No distraction was sufficient. The feeling of doom was so overwhelming that I was truly afraid I might hurt myself. I tried reaching out to friends online, but any comfort they offered was offset by paranoia. I couldn't shake the feeling that somehow this whole benzo thing, the websites, and support groups were all a ruse, part of some grand conspiracy designed to deceive me. I would tell myself that was crazy and look for a distraction from my psychosis. On many such occasions, I would go into the piano room, pick up *Unbroken* from off the bookshelf and hold it to my chest. As I did, I would pace around in circles, telling myself over and over, "if he can do it, I can do it. If he can go on to live a good life, so can I. He can do it, I can do it, I can do it …" I willed myself to stay alive. I looked forward to the day when I could meet Louis in heaven and thank him for being my inspiration.

Four years later, I sat in a dark theater with Paul, watching the previews that played before the movie started. This was a good night. We'd had a good meal, and I was mostly symptom-free that day, just a few aches and pains. Sitting next to my husband, my hand in his, I was content to forget about the world outside for a few hours. Suddenly an unexpected preview for *Unbroken: Path to Redemption* (part two of Louis Zamperini's story) flashed across the 20-foot screen in front of me. Images of Louie struggling with the trauma and recovery from his life-changing experience were transformed as my mind superimposed the footage of my own harrowing memories. I saw me pacing around in the dark, night after night, pleading with myself to hang on, to keep going, begging on my knees for angels to be with me as they were for Louie. I relived those darkest of nights when it took every ounce of strength I had not to take my own life. Tears streamed down my face as I realized those images were a part of my healing journey too. They were tears of both gratitude and pain. Paul, vigilant as ever, noticed my silent sobbing and whispered in my ear, "are you ok?" "I'm fine," I whispered back, "it just ... brings up a lot of memories." He put his arm around me, and I laid my head on his shoulder. I let out a peaceful sigh as the preview of the redemption of Louis Zamperini came to an end.

After his ordeal, Louis Zamperini found God and dedicated the rest of his life to helping others.

I could relate to that.

CHAPTER 16

Born Again

Yet a part of you still believes you can fight and survive no matter what your mind knows. It's not so strange. Where there's still life, there's still hope. What happens is up to God.

LOUIS ZAMPERINI, DEVIL AT MY HEELS

I completed my diazepam taper on June 25, 2015. My husband, the kids, and even Dan and Delores were present that day. They stood around the kitchen counter as I commemorated my final dose of 0.2 mg by breaking my tapering jar with a hammer. After that, we danced around to George Michael's "Freedom." I documented it all on video and uploaded it to my channel. I looked like I felt better than I did. But that's ok. The point was to give hope to others.

At first, I noticed very little difference now that I wasn't taking a benzo every day. In some ways, I felt more stable without the ups and downs of diazepam as it coursed in and out of my veins. But my sleep got worse. This scared me, and for a split second, I considered taking a "rescue dose" to help me sleep. Instantaneously, I remembered everything I had learned and labored to teach others over the past year. I quickly came to myself. No, I would never put another tranquilizer in my mouth again. I relished the idea of no longer agonizing over scheduling and driving to doctor's appointments every month to get my prescription renewed. No more begging, shaming or explaining. No more late-night trips to the 24-hour Walgreens several towns over because I had forgotten to fill my script in time and didn't want to risk a seizure or a trip to the ER. I was no longer a slave to anyone or anything, and that was worth any sacrifice.

Part of the price I paid was pain. Now that the benzo bandage had been ripped from my flesh, I felt all the physical aches and pains it masked throughout my taper. It was nothing like the pain I experienced when withdrawing too fast, but it was surprising to suddenly feel the full bite of my lingering injury in all those muscles and joints. I worried the numbness the medication provided caused me to unwittingly adhere to a daily schedule of light exercise over the past 13 months, which may have actually aggravated my condition. Did a strict regimen of daily exercise help me or hurt me? It's hard to say.

There were lots of little fears like this as I navigated my way out of benzoland, but mostly I had hope. The taper had worked. While feeling hardly any different off the drug was definitely anticlimactic, it was also reassuring. It meant that bits of me had healed as I removed almost imperceptible amounts of the poison day by day. Not feeling any different off the benzo meant I had managed to get to such a small dose that my body hardly perceived its absence. Of course, the diazepam wasn't immediately gone from my body. With a half-life of 50 to 200 hours, it would take about a week for it to work its way out. Given what I have read in research, along with my personal experience and what I have seen in support groups, many of us do not metabolize these drugs properly in the first place, and it's likely that the substance remained in my system for many weeks and possibly even months afterward. Nevertheless, I slowly began to improve.

I remember the first time I cracked a joke. Paul and I were heading out on one of our ritual date nights when I made some wry comment in response to something he had said. I didn't realize anything significant had happened until I saw his eyes. Paul just had this look on his face of adulation and surprise, as though he had suddenly seen me for the first time in years. I sheepishly turned away from his gaze. I felt unworthy of such admiration, for something so unintentional on my part.

Many date nights later, I found myself overcome with joy as I realized that the noisy cafeteria we decided to eat at, was not overwhelming to my senses. The bright lights, the loud clatter of pots and pans, even the proximity and chatter of the people next to me in line, all of it seemed normal. Of course, the sudden realization that this was actually a very abnormal way for me to feel in this situation caused the panic to rise in my throat. No big deal, I had learned every possible way to manage anxiety over the past two years. Now that the chemical-induced fear was ebbing, the techniques that proved useless during my taper were surprisingly effective. I remember another first for me as I stood in line at the grocery market, a year or two after tapering, and actually thought to make small talk with the woman behind me. I smiled at her, made eye contact, and joked about something or other. It felt great! I was exuberant over my little accomplishment.

These breakthroughs weren't like mile markers on a hike towards the summit of recovery. They were more like buoys in the fluctuating whirlpool of rebirth. Whenever I felt myself being sucked back under the vortex of nasty symptoms, I could say to myself, "I reached that marker once before. I'll get there again." Ring by swirling ring, I slow-ly inched farther and farther away from the turbulent epicenter of the benzo abyss, but the maelstrom was infinitely larger than anyone could have guessed.

My injury was more extensive than I realized. Just as I would celebrate shattering through one window, my eyes would land on a previously unseen thick pane of glass up ahead. However, as count-less problems eased or went away, I found I could pick out individual symptoms more accurately. This meant I could actually define them, name them, talk about them, and potentially treat them, which was practically impossible before. There is a freedom that comes with having the language to tell your own story. I continued to share my expanding narrative with my ever-growing number of YouTube fol-lowers, along with friends and family. Hearts were softened, and the understanding I so desperately sought for years suddenly surfaced. It was amazing how much being understood and believed contributed to my healing.

As I continued to improve, I was also more capable of putting on a good face. It was a pleasant deceit that often backfired on me. Paul oozed frustration night and day as I perpetually failed to perform the tasks he thought I should. Occasionally, the dam would burst:

"You care more about your benzo cause than about your own fam-ily!" He would berate. "I need help! I have to go to job sites and meet with clients, and I need someone to do the paperwork!"

On other occasions, Paul chastised me for not following through with the simplest of tasks.

"You can make YouTube videos, but you can't spend 20 min-utes looking up a place for us to go for spring break? Just go to these websites, find something, make a plan. Why do I have to do everything?!"

I would quietly submit to his anger out of guilt for all those many months he single-handedly carried our family on his shoulders. I forgave him because he had already forgiven me for that time I chucked a glass jar at his head with every intention of breaking one or the other. Benzo rage can be nasty, and I guessed I deserved a bit of my own back at me after everything I had put him through. Besides, I couldn't keep my brain and body calm, and also think of an explanation as to why I was still not accomplishing much more on any given day than I had during my taper.

It wasn't until I had healed enough to reflect on my situation and organize my thoughts into spoken words that I calmed the storm one day as I replied to Paul on the phone:

"I know I seem better, and I am. But I'm not as well as you want me to be. I know I'm not doing much, but at least now I can do it without constant suffering. If I push myself too hard, I'm in misery. If I take it slow, life is bearable. If I spend 20 to 40 minutes on the computer, my brain will hurt for the rest of the day, and I won't be able to help Nathaniel and Lucy with their homework when they get home from school. I have to save my brain for the afternoons when I need to read teacher handouts and discuss problems with classmates. I've spent so long suffering. I don't have the willpower to intentionally create more just so I can do some housecleaning or paperwork. I know I'm talking and acting more normal, but I still have a hard time reading and interpreting things. Planning something like a vacation is still beyond me right now. I'm sorry. Please be patient with me. Believe me; I want to do all those things too. I want to help you; to show you how much I love you, how grateful I am for you. I feel guilty every day that I can't. I'm so sorry you still have to do so much."

Tears erupted, as they do so easily these days, and Paul was forgiving. He let go of many of his hopes and expectations for the present. Ironically, in some ways, it was just as difficult for my husband to let go of his additional responsibilities once I did become well enough to take care of them. I would have to tell him over and over, "It's ok. I got this." I couldn't do everything, but I could remember to schedule an appointment or get the kids to practice on time, and if I couldn't, I was rational enough to ask a friend for help.

The kids felt the effects of my recovery a bit differently. At first, they were happy to have mom back in so many little ways. At seven years old, Lucy saw me sit down and play a concert piano piece for the first time in her life. I laughed a little more and talked some more and spent less time hiding from them in my room out of guilt when I wasn't feeling well. Mom was back. But soon they started to realize that, "Uh-oh, mom is back!" It was no longer ok to play video games for hours on end. Yes, making your bed is a real thing. Don't say crap. Watching everything that daddy wants to watch on TV isn't always appropriate. Parents kiss, get used to it.

I could see the humor in all of it. But I was also frustrated with my progress. Other people who had finished their tapers were healing exponentially faster than me. Some were already back working part-time and full-time jobs. I still had a hard time getting through three hours of church on Sunday. But even though my body was bound by limitations, my spirit finally, finally broke free.

The first inkling I had that I might still be connected to God was while sitting in church during a fast and testimony meeting. This must have been when I was near the end of my taper, or just after. As I watched various members of the congregation walk up to the pulpit and talk about their faith in God, their belief in the restoration of The Church of Jesus Christ and his prophets and apostles, I wished that I could join them. Like so many Sundays before, I wished I could say I believed those things, that I was as certain of the truth now as I used to be. But I didn't feel anything anymore. I didn't know anything. I said a silent prayer, "Please, I want to know!" Then the thought entered my mind, "Talk about what you do know."

I was confused. "What do I know?" Memories came to me of pivotal spiritual experiences I'd had in my life, which had been the foundation of my faith. I recalled the time in high school when I was sixteen years old, and I bore my testimony to my friend, Gary, after weeks of praying and fasting on his behalf. He had been going through a spiritual crisis, and I really wanted to help him find the peace I had found in the gospel of Jesus Christ. But, even though I attended seminary for an hour every morning before school and read the scriptures every night before bed, I still wasn't sure if I knew that Jesus Christ was really a living person and really who I believed him to be. After many doctrinal debates with my friend, often in the middle of our social studies class, I finally decided to follow the advice of my seminary teacher (who also happened to be my father), stop wrestling with the facts, and let the Holy Ghost bear witness instead.

I stopped in the middle of a crowded hallway, as hundreds of students hurried past us on their way to their next class, and turned to look Gary square in the face. I didn't know if I could tell him the things I knew he needed to hear because I wasn't sure of them myself, but I decided to take a leap of faith and say them anyway. "I know that Jesus

Christ is my brother and that he lives and loves us ..." I don't remember what I said after that. All I know is that I felt a flame like white fire ignite in the center of my soul, rush out the bottom of my feet and fill me past the top of my head. Then it reached out of my mouth, crossed the space between us, and touched Gary. At that moment I knew, more than I had ever known anything, that Gary felt it too. He opened his mouth and the words, "I know, you know that," came out. Yes, I did. I'd never known anything with more certainty before in my life.

More memories came to mind. I remembered praying desperately for some confirmation that my son Ethan still existed somewhere nearby after his passing, and I remembered the burning in my bosom I experienced in the temple a couple of months later, another witness of the Holy Ghost. I remembered how my first seeds of hope were planted more than 20 years earlier when a kind man took the time to sit with me after a fireside and help me find my way out of the darkness.

As I sat in the back of the chapel, contemplating these memories, my heart began to pound. Not in an anxious way, but rather in a way that I felt compelled to stand, walk past the entire congregation to the front of the church, step behind the microphone, face everyone (boils and all) and bear my testimony. I spoke of how it all started with the speaker who encouraged me that night at youth conference so many years ago to start reading the scriptures every day. I spoke about Gary and Ethan. I ended by saying that I did not know all things, but that I knew these things were true, they really happened, and that I was supposed to share them with the people sitting in the congregation that day. Then I ended in the name of Jesus Christ and walked back to my seat.

After that, I could read the scriptures again. I mean, really sit and read and study and ponder them, and feel inspiration instead of panic. I decided to reread the Book of Mormon from cover to cover. I had done this many times since my youth, and I honestly worried it would be mundane. But it was as if I were reading it for the first time. After all, I was a different person now. Every verse spoke to me, every word related to my situation. I was inspired by the gospel of Jesus Christ. The conduit to God was once again open as light flooded through the shattered opaque glass that had separated me from him. I was no longer cut off from myself. I knew who I was. I was a child of God. I still had to deal with the frustrations and limitations of my circumstances. But I was no longer bound by them. I was free, and as my spirit took flight, I could view my life from a higher perspective. And from this heavenly advantage, I found that peace, "which passeth all understanding." (Philippians 4:7)

It was a wonder that I could have such joy and peace on my good days, in between the bad days. One day, I felt plunged into the depths of an ocean of benzo waves. The next, I was filled with hope for better days to come and a love and desire to reach out and help those around me with my renewed spiritual energy. Sometimes it still felt like this might be it, the wave that never abates, the one that will continue to surge until the end of my days. The door to hell cracked open, and I recalled its heat with perfect clarity. But the one constant in this life is change. Things always change, and with God, it's usually for the better. The waves roll back, his light illuminates the shores of my mind, and I have what I call "my perfect days." These are the days when my mind is clear, and I am productive, despite my pain and fatigue. It's literally like a light is switched on in my brain. When that light is present, I feel joy. No amount of physical symptoms, concerns for my family, our business, or the world around me can overcome it. Even when I feel sadness or anxiety, it's nothing compared to the peace that is my constant companion. I love my perfect days. And when, for whatever reason, the light switch flips off, I know the light is still there, and I look for it with hope in my heart until it returns. I forgive myself for not being perfect on these days because God has already forgiven me, and because I was never really perfect to begin with.

My good days now are practically limitless. I have little to no pain. I'm still finding parts of my brain that I didn't know were asleep, are waking up. It's a tightrope walk to be sure, doing all the things a mom, wife, and activist needs to do while nursing a fragile nervous system. But somehow there are always new answers to new problems that pop up as my brain shifts and my body heals. Sometimes those answers take longer than I would like to unearth. But eventually they find their way to the surface of my mind, and I am reminded of the goodness of God in delivering me from hell. I am reminded of Alma who, after being racked with the endless torment of a damned soul, said: Yea, I say unto you, my son, that there could be nothing so exquisite and so bitter as were my pains. Yea, and again I say unto you, my son, that on the other hand, there can be nothing so exquisite and sweet as was my joy. Alma Ch 36: v21, Book of Mormon

Like Alma, I couldn't have imagined as a teenager the pain I would experience in losing my baby at the age of twenty-five. And I wasn't capable in my twenties of even fathoming the kind of suffering I would endure in my thirties. But with each submersion into dark waters came rebirth. Yes, there are familiar parts of me coming back to life, but I will never be the same person again. That's a good thing.

I realize now that the answer to my prayer, years ago, when I first began my benzo taper, is still being revealed. The prophet Lehi, who was teaching his son when he said, "it must needs be, that there is an opposition in all things" goes on to talk about how this makes us free and says "Adam fell that men might be; and men are, that they might have joy." Joy, freedom ... from opposition? I think I understand now. It's not a tug of war between bad and good where the winner takes all. It's a beautiful harmony, a dance between creation and destruction. Just as there are infinite opportunities for pain and suffering in this life, there is also infinite greatness to be found by embracing the fall into darkness.

Before I was like a lovely vase, pleasing to the eye, but only able to hold so much water. I suppose some vases are deeper than others, and some break more easily, but I believe the master sculptor has a grander vision for each of us than to be receptacles for stagnant water. He says, "For behold, this is my work and my glory — to bring to pass the immortality and eternal life of man."[1] At first, life broke my outer vessel. Choosing God's grace, I allowed him to reform me. Bound together by sturdier stuff I thought I had changed, but I was still a vase. Then I was shattered, pulverized to dust. Consumed by the deluge and washed away until there was nothing left of me to recognize, I cried for an escape from the ocean of my pain. But now I know, fighting to get away from the ocean is pointless. I am the ocean. The creator of worlds without end formed me from the dust into something so deep and so wide it can hold vast seas of both joy and pain. With the help of my Heavenly Father, I will increase even after this life until one day, like him, I span the expanse of eternity.

---

1   Book of Moses 1:39

CHAPTER 17

The Prodigal Son

When you've suffered a great deal in life, each additional pain is both unbearable and trifling.

YANN MARTEL, LIFE OF PI

December 2015,

It's been four months since the As Prescribed *interview and the non-linear beast of healing continues to ravenously eat away at my hope. I spent the last year and a half expecting the reward for all my pain and patience would be to gradually slip back into normalcy. Not so. I had a month or two of false hope, feeling ever so slightly better, only to fall back under the roiling waters of the abyss. I put on a brave face for my two-month post-taper update video on You-Tube, expecting that this was probably just a bad wave and it would soon pass. Two months have turned into four and now five and still no improvement. Was it all a lie? Have I given thousands of online viewers false hope?*

Not long after that journal entry, I read the post of a benzo friend of mine who lamented that after a year of what felt like healing, she had a major setback. Disabled by the severe return of insomnia, among other things, she decided to drastically overhaul her diet. A short time later, she wrote a new post, joyously exclaiming how she had escaped the clutches of her awful wave through nutrition. I was both happy for her and disheartened. I had tried many diets before my injury. I knew how to prepare paleo, vegan, raw vegan, and cultured foods. I had tried them all to see if anything could help, but nothing worked. Once again, it seemed like all the knowledge and learning I had collected fell useless at my feet. What more could I do?

Then I remembered a few of my other friends who were on the other side of healing who had also mentioned following strict diets. They had all recommended seeing a functional medicine doctor or FND. I wasn't familiar with functional medicine. I wondered if it was similar to all the other naturopathic specialists I had seen over the past couple years, the results of which had been disappointing at best. I messaged one of these friends and asked for her help as my benzo brain was making it difficult for me to do a productive online search for a local practitioner. A few minutes later, she sent me a link to the only licensed FND sho could find in Utah, Dr. Jones. The waiting list to get in to see him was usually long, but I lucked out, and got in to see him within a few weeks.

I sat there at my first visit, experiencing not only the pain and disorientation that were my constant companions, but also sweaty and anxious with the anticipation of yet another medical encounter where I had to defend myself against a barrage of condescending comments that lacked even a basic understanding of the pharmacology of the drugs that had harmed me. I gave Dr. Jones a quick "Hi" as he entered the room and did my best to make normal human eye contact for half a second. After that, I stared at the jade-green tiles on the wall next to the bamboo plant. Practically bulging out of his smock due to his broad shoulders and stout frame, the FND didn't come across as particularly friendly.

Bypassing any small talk, Dr. Jones went straight for the examination. I answered all his questions, explaining how I had recently completed a painfully long taper and what symptoms I was still experiencing. He responded by explaining how benzodiazepines interrupt the GABA/glutamate cycle and perpetuate the vicious cycle of less and less GABA for various metabolic processes. I had already learned about this, but not in such detail. His understanding encouraged me, and I opened up some more. I told him about the severity of my cognitive disability, and he nonchalantly explained that physical stress on the body makes you "stupid." "Oh, I almost forgot," I said towards the end of the interview, "I was also floxed twice on Cipro." As I prepared to define the term floxed for him, Dr. Jones's mask of dispassionate professionalism gave way to a look of shock that surprised me. He was the first doctor who acted like my problems were as big as I knew they were. He redirected the conversation to address any physical problems I may have been experiencing from the exposure to fluoroquinolones.

Although I found it very difficult to adequately answer all his questions or even to remember what symptoms I did and didn't have, this was by far the most productive conversation I'd ever had with any doctor I had encountered in the past five years. When I told him that I was wary of certain treatments he recommended, due to my extreme sensitivity, he changed course without batting an eye to offer alternative methods. The most important thing Dr. Jones stressed during our visit was diet. Not only did he prescribe for me a high protein diet to treat the insulin imbalance and muscle deterioration caused by the benzos, but he also gave me a gut reset diet protocol to follow over the first few weeks. This was to treat the painful "benzo belly" I had described to him, which made my abdomen feel rock hard and had me looking like I was three to four months pregnant. He also told me I was dehydrated and gave me a recipe for a homemade electrolyte mix to be taken with 32 ounces of water at least once a day.

I couldn't believe how much understanding I received in that 45-minute consultation! I felt hopeful as I walked up to the front office to plunk down a considerable amount of cash for the appointment, and to schedule the blood work for my next visit. I read over the protocol and diet guidelines. I would have to strictly measure out my daily fat, protein, and carbohydrate intake. 150 grams of pure protein seemed like a lot, but Dr. Jones assured me I would lose seven to eight pounds if I did it right. That sounded great to me. Ever since the end of my taper, I had been steadily gaining unwanted weight. I was willing to do whatever it took to get better.

It took less than a week of diet and supplements to see the seeds of my hope finally bear fruit. Within days I was sleeping seven to eight hours every night. I could think, talk, read. I went from 30 percent functionality to 60 percent. It was December, and we were preparing to take the family to Las Vegas over the Christmas break to visit Grandma and Grandpa. For the first time in years, I packed all our bags.

When we got to the rambler off Nellis and Sahara in the heart of downtown Las Vegas, I got out of the car to stretch out my painful lower back and neck. I could barely stand upright at first, but I felt great. A little body pain and stiffness was nothing compared to the brain pain I used to have. My depersonalization and derealization were now only mild annoyances. Dan and Delores remarked on the difference in my countenance. It was the first Christmas since 2012 that I actually enjoyed.

After we came back to Utah, I went through some old messages and found a few from some friends who had encouraged me to audition for a musical play they were in called *The Prodigal Son*. Initially, I despaired at the invitation, unwilling to explain to them how impossible a task that would be for me. Now, I wanted to do this more than anything. Paul encouraged me and helped me set up our camera. The date for sending in my audition video had already passed, but I figured I'd be allowed to join the chorus at least. I stood in front of the piano and recorded myself belting out the lyrics to "All That Jazz." I felt so free! My voice, my expressions, my movements, I felt like the me I had hoped was still inside had finally broken out of her prison cell. I felt like a human being again.

The next week I was offered a lead role in the production. Every Saturday I made the drive up to Salt Lake to practice with the choir and orchestra. We blocked out scenes. I offered to fill in for the choreographer when she couldn't come to practice. I choreographed an entire piece by myself for the "Fallen Idol" number. I laughed, I joked, and I breathed through the dizziness and pain whenever they threatened to overwhelm me. I was happy with my new life. It was more perfect than I could have imagined.

Then Nathaniel got sick. It was February, and I was only a month into rehearsals. It wasn't uncommon for the kids to come home with something that was being passed around at the end of winter. As usual, Lucy got over her cold in a few days. But with Nathaniel, things were rarely that simple. Ever since he was born, he seemed to be more sensitive to life. Foods, emotions, viruses, these things caused him more problems than other kids. I have no doubt that Nathaniel's exposure to Ambien combined with steroids in the womb and subsequent withdrawal after delivery contributed to this condition. Then there were the antibiotics he took for the cryptosporidium he got from the local pool as a toddler and the c-diff he developed soon after. After that, when he'd get something as simple as a common cold, it seemed our little boy just couldn't shake it for weeks, often ending up in the hospital hooked up to an IV due to the dehydration from an uninterrupted week of diarrhea and vomiting. Despite my best efforts to heal his gut through nutrition, Nathaniel continued to have these extreme reactions. But eventually, Nathaniel would get better and go back to being a normal kid.

This time though, it was a head cold that had moved into his chest. No vomiting, no hospitals, so I wasn't too worried about it. An entire life of bad karma with doctors told me just to let his body work it out on its own. Paul, however, took what he believed to be a more cautious approach. He waited with bated breath until the ten-day minimum I required before taking the kids to the pediatrician was up. But I decided not to take Nathaniel to the doctor that week. After another couple of weeks, Paul became really anxious. Nathaniel's cough had lingered for four or five weeks now, and Paul argued for putting our son on an antibiotic. I was against it. Despite my newfound wellness, it was often difficult for me to get through a whole day without lying down to rest or nap. I didn't see the need to wear myself or my son out with a stressful trip to the doctor for a common cold.

On Saturday morning, Paul called a friend of his who was a physician assistant and asked him to call in a prescription for bronchitis.

He picked up the Z-Pack from Walgreens and gave it to Nathaniel the next morning. Soon afterward, Nathaniel started complaining about a tummy ache. We figured the antibiotics were irritating him and asked him to just tough it out at church. Halfway through Sunday school, one of Nathaniel's teachers went to find Paul and brought him to Nathaniel who was curled up in a ball on the floor by the drinking fountain, crying out in pain. Unsure what was wrong, he scooped Nathaniel up and carried him home.

I didn't know about the incident at church, and by the time I got home, Nathaniel was beginning to swell with a rash and a fever. We thought it might be an anaphylactic reaction like the one he'd inexplicably had one day after coming home from a friend's house, but his breathing was ok. Despite the swollen hands, feet, face, and neck, his throat seemed to be unobstructed. Nathaniel was crying out every few minutes with waves of stomach pain, but he didn't vomit or have diarrhea. We gave him some Benadryl and took him to the doctor, but nothing helped. His cracked lips and hands eventually healed, his rash cleared up, but the pain continued to eat away at our son. He couldn't even stand upright. We borrowed a wheelchair from a neighbor and trudged on. Paul insisted we reach out to every possible medical practitioner we could. I felt they would all end up being a big waste of time. But I still didn't trust myself. I knew I was coming from a place of fear, and I knew how bad my decisions were when that was my foundation.

We spent the next few months scheduling appointments with specialists all over the valley. I was grateful just to be somewhat capable of driving my son to these appointments, but every time I had to walk into a doctor's office, I felt a sense of dread as memories of my abuse at the hands of medical professionals flashed in front of my eyes. I had arguments in my head with the doctors as I drove to appointments. I hated going. I hated that we were forced to be dependent on their horrible pharmaceutical system once again. Besides being a waste of time, it was also a waste of money. Nothing came of any of it, as expected, and it seemed like the precious good windows I should have been spending creating new memories with my kids, were wasted debating with doctors. When the bad waves that were an inevitable part of my recovery consumed me, Paul would leave work to take Nathaniel to his next appointment for me.

I felt guilty for my Saturday escapes to *The Prodigal Son* rehearsals. I enjoyed myself too much, even as my back and pelvis flared up from the combination of dancing, carrying Nathaniel up and down the stairs and lifting his frail but lengthy body in and out of a wheelchair every day. I discussed quitting the play with Paul and asked him for a blessing of comfort and guidance. He laid his hands on my head and told me words I did not expect to hear. I was told my Heavenly Father was proud of me for how well I had endured my trials. He told me I was helping many of his children, and this play was an opportunity he desired for me, that it would be a blessing to others. He told me I would have the strength both to see it through and help my son. I sat in awe. Then, reassured by that blessing, I went to rehearsals.

Meanwhile, a battery of tests showed Nathaniel had eosinophilic esophagitis. It explained some of his sensitivities, but not the relentless, debilitating stomach pain that had made our once rambunctious son bedridden. The pediatric allergist I spoke to, the best in the valley according to friends, denied that the newly diagnosed EOE could have been caused by the interaction with the azithromycin our son had taken. "EOE is something you're born with. You don't suddenly

develop it." Really? I thought. Because our son was walking and running around, drinking gallons of milk the day before, and the day after
he can't walk or eat cereal. But I didn't say that.

I tried to show him the recent black box warning the FDA put out
about azithromycin and the interaction between it and persons with
EOE. The black box notification was posted in my fluoroquinolone
support group barely a few weeks after Nathaniel's interaction. "It
says they develop DRESS,[1] which is exactly what happened to him;
he had all the symptoms they describe. This could have caused his
EOE." "He didn't have DRESS," the expert declared, "If he'd had that
he would have died." I had a hard time pulling up the article on my
phone. I had a hard time seeing straight that afternoon. I just knew
that this is what happened to my son and nobody believed me except
the internet.

Doctor after doctor confirmed what I already knew. When they
don't understand a problem, they throw psychiatric drugs at it. Despite the recent black box warning advising against it, our son was
prescribed opiates and benzos in combination. We didn't give him the
benzos, but we gave the opiates a try; they just made him worse. They
offered us tricyclic antidepressants and SSRIs. The doctors were un-
concerned about his genetic predisposition for adverse reactions to

---

1   DRESS syndrome (Drug Rash with Eosinophilia and Systemic Symptoms) is an adverse reaction
    term that is currently used to describe a hypersensitivity reaction with an estimated mortality of
    up to 10% ... It is a severe, idiosyncratic multisystem reaction to a drug, characterized by fever,
    skin rash, lymphadenopathy, haematological abnormalities and internal organ involvement.
    Prescriber Update 32(2): 12-13
    June 2011
    http://www.medsafe.govt.nz/profs/PUArticles/DRESSsyndromeJune2011.htm

serotonergic drugs. One doctor told us he thought Nathaniel was having stomach migraines and offered us "migraine medication." It was a bipolar med. Too bad they didn't read their own literature. They would have seen the drugs they were offering our son put him at risk for another bout of DRESS. Each time I refused their suggested treatments, I was treated with disdain. We were labeled noncompliant. I even had one doctor, an infectious disease specialist, yell at me and stomp out of the room, leaving Nathaniel and me sitting across from his baffled intern, because I didn't want to give my son psychiatric medications. I couldn't imagine why he should care so much if my son took psych meds or not; he wasn't even prescribing them to Nathaniel. But I was used to this by now; it was nothing new.

Once again, Paul and I were required to question everything we knew. Our son was in pain. He couldn't eat. He'd lost so much weight I would cry when I saw him without a shirt on, his pelvic bones jutting out like an old photo of a concentration camp victim. Maybe we should just give him something, anything to ease the pain. We tried steroids. One made him worse right away, and the other made him better for a month until it made him worse. At our wit's end, we considered moving to Colorado on the chance that medical marijuana might bring Nathaniel some relief from the day and night waves of pain that made him cry out every five to ten minutes. As a last-ditch effort, Paul found a local CBD company. CBD is a compound of cannabis that is legal to sell in Utah. We brought some home for Nathaniel and put several drops under his tongue that night. The next morning, he awoke to waves of pain that had spread out to every 15 to 20 minutes. Then it was a half-hour and then an hour.

We ditched the specialists and made an appointment with Dr.

Jones, my FND. His allergy testing showed something totally different from the pediatric allergist's, which basically said Nathaniel was now allergic to everything. Dr. Jones explained why that test would show that and why it was inaccurate. He recommended a specific diet and some supplements to help with the inflammation. We hoped and prayed this would finally help our son.

There's a picture of our family standing in front of the Conference Center at Temple Square after one of my performances of *The Prodigal Son*, me in costume, Nathaniel in his wheelchair. He is smiling. We're all smiling, another miracle considering how my body fell apart the last couple of weeks before the performances. My voice had started cracking again, and the shift to nightly rehearsals made it difficult for me to sleep. Between that and the resurgence of severe pelvic pain, I had to start faking my way through my songs. The more I did that, the more self-conscious I became. It was a vicious cycle of fatigue and anxiety that all came to a head the last two nights of dress rehearsal when some cast members found me choking in the dressing room. Still a common symptom for me, I would suddenly have that sensation you get when something goes down the wrong pipe, and you can't breathe for a minute. I had learned to stay calm and focus as soon as the wheezing started. The calmer I remained, the sooner it would usually pass. The other cast members were freaking out, asking if I was having an asthma attack or if they needed to call an ambulance. I couldn't answer, of course. I just shook my head as I sat on the floor and held up my hand as if to say, "hold on a minute." After the episode passed and I could talk again, I told my friend in my raspy voice that this was a common part of my condition and assured her I would be ok. She was still very concerned and asked if she could get one of the male cast members to give me a blessing. I agreed.

As I sat alone on the floor of the dressing room, I began to question the sanity of three performances in two days with a son at home languishing from an iatrogenic illness and myself, just barely a few months into recovery from my own. Stephanie came back into the dressing room with Larry, the president of a Spanish branch of The Church of Jesus Christ in Salt Lake. Exhausted, I got up and sat in a chair as he placed his hands on my head. Astoundingly, but not surprisingly, Larry repeated to me the very words my husband had said to me months before on the night I had asked him for a blessing. I was told the lord was proud of me for being so strong, of how much I had helped others, how he wanted me to do this play and that I would be able to do it. I thanked Larry and drove home, convinced I could do this.

The next morning, I had to ask the mother of a young cast member to drive me up to Salt Lake as I was too weak to drive myself. Just before the first performance, I asked another male cast member to give me a blessing. I hadn't slept much that week, and I was in a bad wave. I just couldn't imagine going out on stage in my condition. For a third time, the same words of the same blessing were repeated to me. I walked out on that stage, believing I could do it. I made it through all three performances. I even went outside to mingle with audience members after each show. Then I would lie down in a dark room doing deep breathing until it was time for the next performance or mic check.

In the months following my final performance, Nathaniel slowly continued to improve. Even better, he was putting on weight! He never really finished his third-grade year of school even though I was officially "homeschooling" him. He had been too sick to do more than watch educational shows on TV. But by the fall of 2016, we had en-rolled him in an online homeschool program which I endeavored to teach despite the breakdown of my body over the past few months. Nathaniel and I toiled through the pain and cog fog until the carpool brought Lucy home from school, and we could rest. Eventually, we made it out to some field trips. We worked together on our first science fair project, creating mini hovercrafts to demonstrate air pressure and friction. Paul had to step in and help with that one since I had never done a science project of my own growing up. I was also becoming in-creasingly distracted by the returning neuralgia in my face and neck. Pushing through the pain sapped more and more energy from me. Lucy, however, was full of energy and more than happy to assist in testing different materials on various surfaces.

Our little family had come so far, and yet it seemed like we were going backward in so many ways. A knee injury now aggravated Paul's back and neck injuries. He was always in pain; I was in pain; our son was in pain. When would there be a respite from all this pain? I was still very grateful for every perfect day. But they seemed to be fewer and further apart. I knew I was better even on my worst days now than when I was in withdrawal. It wasn't that my bad days were so awful so much as the frustration of knowing a good day was unbearably close, just an hour or a day or an undiscovered supplement away. It made waiting intolerable.

CHAPTER 18

Fruits of Hope

Broken minds can be healed just the way broken hearts and broken bones are healed ... I bear witness of that day when loved ones whom we knew to have disabilities in mortality will stand before us glorified and grand, breathtakingly perfect in body and mind. What a thrilling moment that will be! I do not know whether we will be happier for ourselves that we have witnessed such a miracle or happier for them that they are fully perfect and finally "free at last."

JEFFREY R. HOLLAND, LIKE A BROKEN VESSEL

Fall 2016

My favorite time of year is fall. I love going for a drive when the air is crisp despite the brilliance of the desert sun in a cloudless cobalt sky. There's something about getting into a sun-warmed car and going for a drive, having to roll down the windows because the air inside is toasty, and feeling the cool breeze on my face, that's just deliciously soothing to my soul.

On one such fall day, while Lucy was still at school, I had Nathaniel join me out on the front porch. Despite the good days, he'd spent a lot of time over the past year lying on the couch, in pain. It was a daily challenge to navigate his illness while pushing past my own limitations and still effectively homeschool my son. Today it wasn't worth it to make ourselves both sick with schoolwork. I scooped up my 9-year-old's emaciated 50-pound body, blanket and all, and carried him out the front door to where our big wooden rocking chair sat. He was too big to fit comfortably in my lap, but I held him just the same. I was grateful they weren't cutting the hay today in the horse pasture across the road. Bringing Nathaniel outside during the harvest season was a bit of an allergy minefield, which I tried to avoid. Today I figured it was worth the risk to get him some much needed fresh air and sunshine. My toes barely reached the cement as I rocked in the oversized chair, back and forth, back and forth.

"Mommy, what if I'm not able to ever go on a mission or go to college? I don't think I could do that."

I kept rocking. I thought about the things that inspired me to keep trying, like the story of Louis Zamperini.

"Do you know where you come from, who your ancestors are?"

He looked up at me.

"You have a great heritage. Your great-grandpa, Poppy, didn't learn English until he went to school. He grew up on a farm in Colorado, and every year, he'd start school late because he was needed at the end of summer to help with the harvest. Then, in the spring, he had to leave school early to help with the planting. He would have to catch up in the fall and work ahead in the winter so he could complete his studies. Your grandpa graduated valedictorian of his high school. He enlisted early on in WWII. He was so smart they wanted him to go to training to become a commissioned officer, even though he was Hispanic, but he thought it was smarter to stay as he was and lead his men as a sergeant. His men trusted and loved him.

"Poppy told me about this one time when he had his men tie up a corporal who had ordered them to attack a town that was occupied by German soldiers. It was towards the end of the war, and the officer was young and inexperienced. Poppy said he didn't have enough men and it would have been a death sentence. Livid, the young commander threatened to court-martial your grandpa. Poppy didn't care. Instead, he asked for a volunteer gunman and a translator, he took the jeep and rode into town like he owned the joint. He asked to see the commanding officer. When the commander came out, he gave Poppy a crisp salute. Poppy offered him a careless, sloppy salute in reply to show him how very unimpressed he was with his rank. He told him he had guns, tanks, so many men, and air power at his disposal. He told him to have his soldiers bring all their weapons to the center of town and lay them down. Poppy would accept their surrender. The commander was hesitant. Just then, an American plane happened to pass them overhead; Poppy pointed to it as if to say 'see.' The soldiers surrendered, and not a single life was lost. Poppy's commanding officer took all the credit, and Poppy was never court-martialed."

I continued my inspirational speech:

"Did you know that when he was in Germany, he was blown up by a landmine? That's when he lost his hearing. He had bits of shrapnel coming out of his body the rest of his life. Poppy was in espionage, and one time he had to go behind enemy lines when he was in the Pacific. Some Japanese soldiers found him. They didn't want to shoot him for fear the American soldiers nearby would hear them, so they took him to a ditch, stabbed him with bayonets and left him for dead. Once he even showed me a small mark on his head where they stabbed his skull. He survived that too. When he got home, he went to barber

SEEDS OF HOPE 179

college then opened his own barber shop. After selling off his business he kept working, helping Uncle Al make stucco coins and traveling to Salt Lake to translate church records almost until the day he died at the ripe old age of 94."

Nathaniel didn't say anything so I went on,

"Your great-grandpa Benji was a bit older and never served in the war, but he was also a very good man. He helped Grandma Lucy escape an abusive marriage and adopted her two boys as his own. It was the great depression, and all they could afford to live in was a shack on a piece of corner property. Year after year, Grandpa Benji added onto the little shack, shored up the walls and the roof and made it into a lovely home. Even though it was the depression, Grandma Lucy said he was never unemployed. He always managed to find work. He ended up working for the Pueblo steel mill, which was hard work and made his lungs sick. But he never complained. When the missionaries taught their family about the word of wisdom, Grandpa Benji decided to quit smoking the next day. Just like that, he put down his cigarettes and never smoked another cigarette, ever again.

"This is who you come from. You have a heritage of great people who have overcome impossible odds. It's in your DNA. You're going to be fine."

"But what if I can't?"

I inhaled and let out a slow, steady breath. It was hard for me to think or talk with my head vibrating as it does on my off days. I said a silent prayer. "Dear Heavenly Father, please give me the words to say …"

I kept on rocking.

"I think you're smart and funny and have an understanding of hardship that most kids your age don't have. Maybe you can use that to help other people someday. But even if you flipped burgers at Mc-Donald's for the rest of your life, that would be ok with me. Because when you came to this earth, there was no requirement saying you had to go to college and earn lots of money. There's no part of the gospel that says you have to be brilliant, or popular, or gorgeous, or famous. The only requirement is that you learn how to be a good person. Every one of us will be resurrected, no matter what. God loves all his children, and he has a glory for each one of us after we die. Now, if you want to live with God after this life, then you also need to get baptized and receive the holy ghost by the laying on of hands. If you want to be exalted and live with your family forever, then you'll need to go through the temple too. That's it. You've already been baptized, and when you're ready, you'll be endowed in the temple. After that, all you're asked to do is endure. Even if for some reason you couldn't do those things, other good people could do them for you in the temple after you leave this life. God has provided a way for everyone in every situation. So, basically, if you can just get through this life and still end up being a good person, then you've succeeded."

I felt the profound silence that follows a moment of truth, and I knew Nathaniel felt it too. We continued to rock for a while longer, feeling the warm sun on our cool cheeks.

Back and forth, back and forth.

Nathaniel successfully finished a full year of homeschool by the next spring, and just as the school year ended, we welcomed a new addition to our family. She came by plane after we received a call from an old friend who asked us if we had a room to spare for a few weeks for a girl from his ward in Ecuador. Genesis was coming to Utah to go to school and needed a place to stay until the apartment she contracted to rent became available for the summer.

Cherubic of face and similar in nature, Genesis was a returned missionary who had joined the church when she was 12 years old. She saved up all her money to serve a mission in Peru for 18 months. When she turned 20, she returned to Guayaquil to a call to be the relief society president over all the women in her ward. She seemed like an exceptional young woman. But, Genesis had no idea when she came to the US how difficult it was going to be to try to find a job that would pay enough to cover her schooling and rent, especially with the laws that required her to work only on campus with a student visa. There was no campus for her English school, and although the sponsor who brought her here committed on paper to fund her education, in reality, he was never going to be able to do that.

This girl didn't even know how to get a bus pass on her own, much less how to navigate the maze of getting an ID and applying for jobs around town in between classes. She needed help. I was doing pretty well at that time; the neuralgia was at bay, and Nathaniel had improved so much that we had decided to register him at the local public elementary school for the upcoming year. We figured we could share our home and food with someone who needed a leg up. We extended Genesis the invitation to stay with us until her situation was more secure. She readily accepted, and Genesis immediately became a part of our family.

Despite all she had experienced in her 22 years of life in a third world country, Genesis had a zest for life, love, and laughter that was contagious. We on the other hand were still used to living in survival mode. Our new daughter drew us out from behind the wall of sorrow we had constructed around our lives and taught us how to have fun again. Paul and I soon found ourselves on the fast track to learning how to parent a young adult who also needed to catch up on being an American teenager.

Less than a month after the arrival of our Ecuadorian daughter, I had another bad wave. Each meal I ate would cause the pain and inflammation in my neck and head to explode. It was hard to see straight. Talking made my head vibrate, and even my hair was falling out again. What was causing it this time? Thyroid? Anemia? Insulin? As had become my practice, I would have to study, seek counsel, pray, and tweak my diet and supplements until a solution presented itself, which it always did, even if it took longer than I liked.

Meantime, I could usually make it through the day by fasting for two meals. But after the evening meal, I had to rely on my 22-year-old girl to help with the kids and clean up dinner. Genesis joyously did everything she could to seek out ways to help. She lived each moment with pure gratitude for her adopted family. To me, she was a saving angel. We came to realize that we needed Genesis every bit as much as she needed us. Especially Paul. I knew how hard it had been for Paul to see his son lose so much of his ability to do normal kid things like toss a football with his dad or go on camping trips. Nathaniel tried hard, but he still had many problems that waxed and waned in severity, making it frustratingly difficult for him to develop a "normal" father-son relationship and friendships with other boys. It was distressing for me, but even more so, I think, for Paul. Every so often, tears would well up in his eyes as he told me how angry he still was about losing Ethan. "I can't get rid of this sense that our family was supposed to have another child, and that Nathaniel was supposed to have an older sibling. It's so obvious he needs that. It doesn't make sense." He didn't have to say it, but I knew he felt like, once again, God had blessed others in extraordinary ways while he was left to sort it out on his own.

I shed tears of my own for my husband's broken heart. Ethan's passing had eventually brought us closer together, like every other trial we endured, by trusting in the passage of time and God's grace. But I worried this unhealed wound in my husband's soul might fester until it ate away at his relationship with the son that was still living. I didn't realize it at first, but after Genesis came into our home, Paul became less bitter about Nathaniel's situation and rarely mentioned his sorrow regarding Ethan. It wasn't until I gathered the family together for a gospel doctrine lesson that I found out why.

I was so grateful to be having a perfect day that Sunday, so I could be clear minded enough to lead the family in a discussion on the first chapters of Matthew and Luke. One of the themes we explored was the humility of the two women in these verses, Mary and Elizabeth, who were examples of accepting the Lord's blessings in his own time and in his own way. Genesis related to their stories by sharing how frequently and fervently she had prayed all growing up for a father. Genesis had a dad who lived with her and her mother, but he was not kind to them. In her heart, she wished for a father who would love her and tell her he was proud of her. She couldn't understand why the other children around her were blessed with loving dads when she wasn't. Genesis said that one day, after she came to live with us, she was walking out the door on her way to a church fireside when Paul called out, "I'm so proud of you." Months later, in between choking sobs and a waterfall of tears, Genesis managed to tell us how much that meant to her and how Paul had been God's answer to all those years of pleading with the lord to have a father in her life.

I already knew how Genesis felt about Paul, and while her testimony was touching, it came as no surprise to me. Paul's did, though. After she finished, my husband related to our children how he had struggled for more than 15 years with the loss of our first son and the hole it had left in his heart and in our family. He said that when Genesis came into our home, he felt like she had suddenly filled that void. She was the older sibling to our children he knew they needed, providing all the love and guidance and playful companionship they had lacked in the past. Genesis was our daughter in every way that mattered. For Paul, she was the older child he knew had been missing from his life. For me, Genesis was a special reminder of God's love for all his children, proof that his plan is for us to all be loved and to live forever in joy with our families, evidence that if we trust him, he will make sure that happens even if it's not in the ways we expect.

One night, soon after Genesis had been unofficially adopted into our family, she, Nathaniel, and Lucy all came into our bedroom and plopped down on the king-sized bed next to me as I lay there with my head vibrating. Sprawled out on the white down comforter they chatted happily until a box that sat unnoticed for years on our chest of drawers suddenly caught Lucy's eye.

"What's that?" Lucy asked as she jumped up from the bed, pointing at the 12×8 sepia colored box, painted white peace lilies adorning its exterior.

"Nathaniel knows what that is," I told her. I had shown him its contents once or twice over the years.

"I don't remember," Nathaniel said.

I was a little miffed at that, but it probably had more to do with the frustrating pain in my neck and face as I lay propped up on the pillows of my bed.

"Nathaniel, you don't remember? That's Ethan's box."

The kids were well aware of their older brother, who was living with his Heavenly Father. We weren't shy about discussing this with them. We wanted them to know that mommy and daddy being sealed to each other in the temple also meant we were eternally sealed to all of our kids, even the ones on the other side of the veil. Ethan was still just as much a part of our family as if he were here, and the kids spoke of him often.

"Can I see what's inside?" Lucy queried.

"Bring it here, and we can look through it together."

Genesis had a curious look on her face. She knew very little of Ethan, and as Lucy set the box in the middle of the bed, Paul switched from English to Spanish to better explain to her what this was all about. I opened the lid, and all three kids leaned in to have a look. Inside were ultrasound pictures, a lock of hair, footprints and many, many cards and letters written to us by members of our North Carolina ward after the funeral. There were also some pictures of Ethan. I made sure to quickly remove the ones of him in the hospital right after the delivery. I didn't want the kids to see the red muscles exposed through the parts of his delicate blue skin that had torn off. They didn't need to see pictures of my pitiful, swollen, crying face.

Lucy began to rummage through the contents excitedly while Nathaniel held back, a distressed look on his face.

"Lucy, be careful!" he said over and over. Her cavalier attitude made him more and more anxious until he finally stood up and started pacing around the room.

"I just ... I can't handle anymore."

"It's ok," I said. "I understand."

Nathaniel's stomach problems had been accompanied by an explosion of debilitating anxiety. I knew what that felt like and did my best to give him the compassion and understanding he required. I looked at Genesis and braced myself for the questions that would naturally enter her mind as she looked through the photos that were too graphic to allow the younger kids to see. I tried to think of how to translate it all into simple English and the Spanish words I knew. I looked from Genesis to Paul, then from Lucy to Nathaniel, and finally, at what I had of Ethan.

"Was it all worth it?"

I heard the unbidden words enter my mind. The question referred to 16 years of struggle two imperfect people went through to stay married to each other. It was asking how I felt about the sorrow I experienced in losing one son and raising another who has to suffer from the effects of medications that gave him debilitating pain, insomnia, and anxiety. It questioned my feelings on spending more than a year of my life in the worst agony imaginable, unable even to love the children I labored to bring into this world. It asked about caring for a husband through more than a decade of car accidents and back injuries, ER visits, and a miscarriage. Was all of that really worth it, just to have the opportunity to gain a body, for the chance to marry Paul and have these kids and live with them forever — in other words — to be like God?

"Was that even a real question?" I defiantly shot back.

Yes, of course, it was.

Epilogue

What is hope?

Where does it come from?

I've asked myself this many times as I see people I care about suffering in ways I can only imagine. Why do human beings who are born into slavery fight to be free when they've known no other life? Why do others who are held captive by abuse, war, poverty, and illness keep trying, even though there's no earthly reason to do so? This seems to be a pretty universal trait in humankind. Could it be we hope for something higher and better because of a voice inside us which says, *"You're a stranger here,*[1] *there's more to life than the sum of your parts and the brokenness all around you."* What if this sense of worth comes from something divine in each of us, a primal knowledge inherited from before the foundations of the world? What if we're not meant to be comfortable with disease and death because we are destined for perfection and immortality, a divine heritage we naturally seek as literal spirit sons and daughters of our Heavenly Mother and Father?

As with Eve, hope gives us the faith to act, to step into the darkness, one foot in front of the other until we come full circle to the tree of life and light that springs from the fountain of living waters which

---

1   O My Father Hymn 292 LDS Hymnal

is the love of Christ. It's that love we hope for; it's this light we seek even when we don't know how we can keep going on or why we keep trying. Somehow, we find the strength, sometimes minute by minute. The same heavenly strength on which we draw for our daily existence is the same power by which hearts are healed, wrongs are forgiven, and weakness is turned into strength. It's this love that gives us the strength to reach out to others who are suffering and lift them up, even though we're drowning too.

"But why, why must it be so hard?" we ask. I don't know! All I know is that we chose this life, knowing it would be hard — not just hard — impossible. So impossible, in fact, that the only way to make it is if a savior were sent to rescue us from death, from sorrow and from the sins of this world. Maybe when we become so desperate that any hope in our own strength is extinguished and we cry out in the darkness for relief; that's the catalyst for the life inside those seeds of hope we carry to germinate within us, radiating new hope and new life as they reach towards the heavens. That's the miracle of hope! Seeds fertilized by pain and sorrow are transformed by love and light into a garden blossoming forever with the fruits of infinite and eternal joy.

If only we can nourish that hope.

But behold, if ye will awake and arouse your faculties, even to an experiment upon my words, and exercise a particle of faith, yea, even if ye can no more than desire to believe, let this desire work in you, even until ye believe in a manner that ye can give place for a portion of my words.

Now, we will compare the word unto a seed. Now, if ye give place, that a seed may be planted in your heart, behold, if it be a true seed, or a good seed, if ye do not cast it out by your unbelief, that ye will resist the Spirit of the Lord, behold, it will begin to swell within your breasts; and when you feel these swelling motions, ye will begin to say within yourselves—It must needs be that this is a good seed, or that the word is good, for it beginneth to enlarge my soul; yea, it beginneth to enlighten my understanding, yea, it beginneth to be delicious to me...But if ye will nourish the word, yea, nourish the tree as it beginneth to grow, by your faith with great diligence, and with patience, looking forward to the fruit thereof, it shall take root; and behold it shall be a tree springing up unto everlasting life.

Alma 32, Book of Mormon

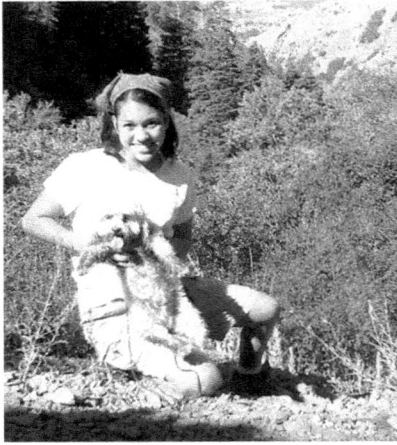

Me and Max after Ethan's passing

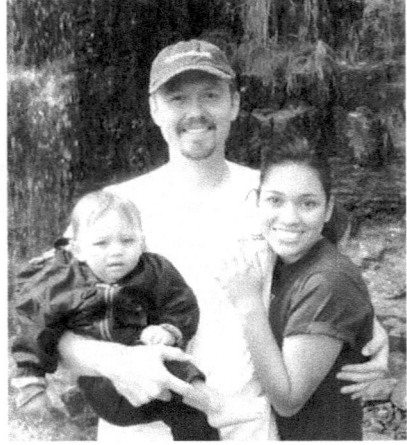

After my c-section and 1st Ambien cold turkey

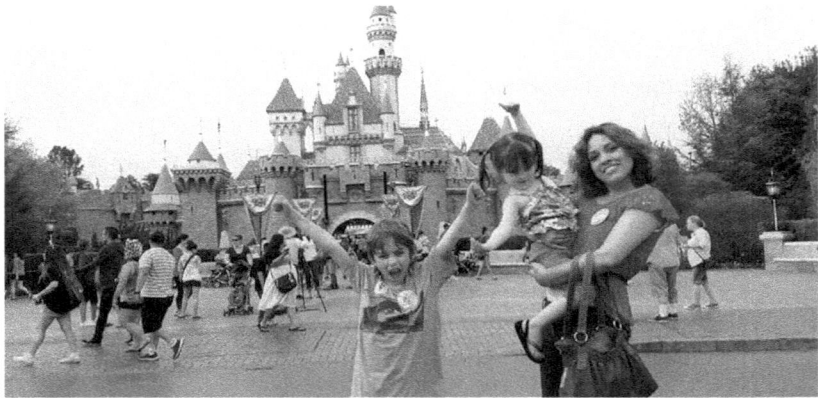

Disneyland trip after miscarriage

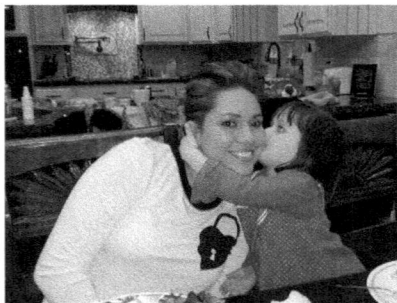

Cymbalta withdrawal

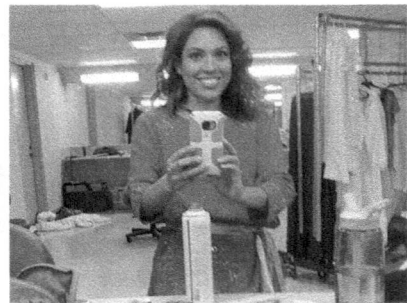

The Prodigal Son dress rehearsal

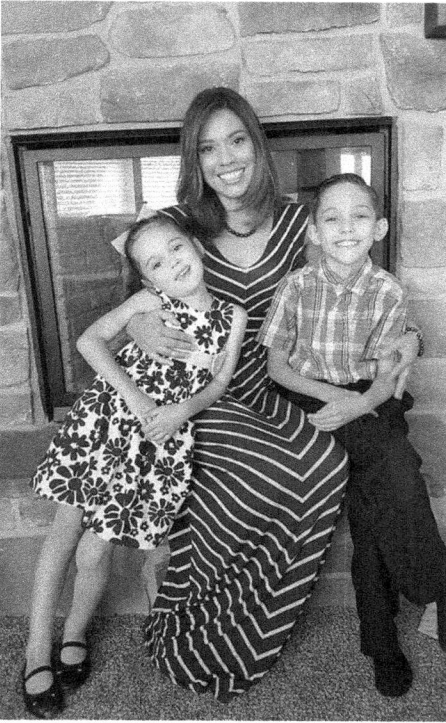

One year after my benzo taper

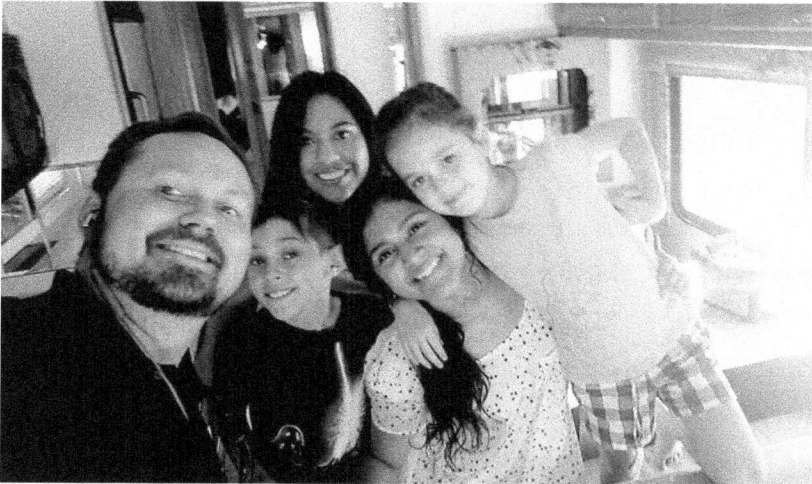

Genesis joins the family

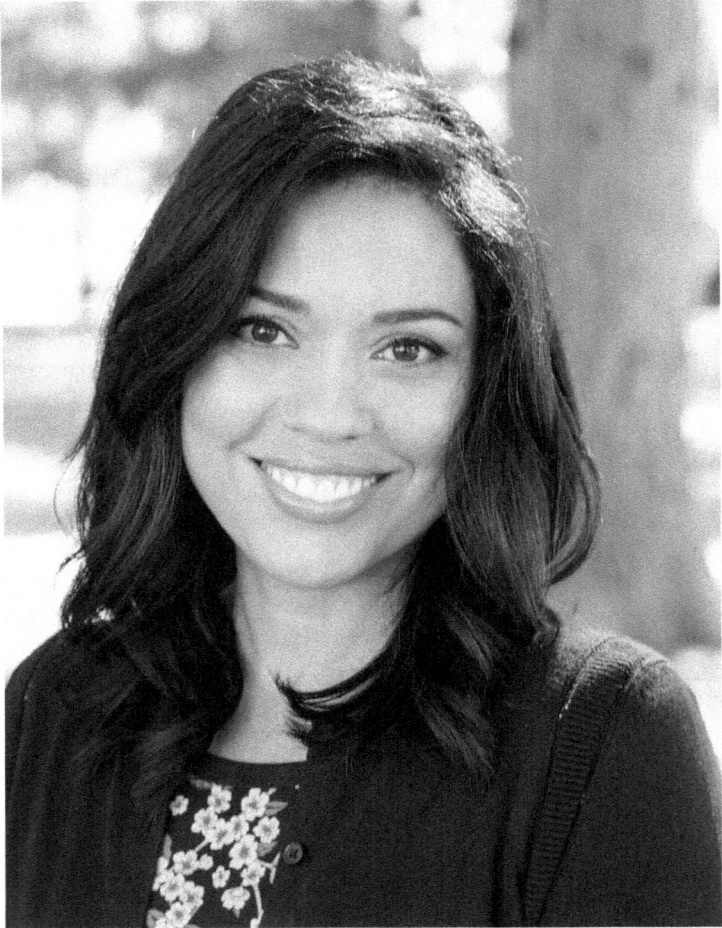

Jocelyn Pedersen is a graduate of Brigham Young University. She grew up in Pueblo, Colorado and now lives with her husband and children in American Fork, Utah. When she's not busy managing her Benzo Brains YouTube channel or serving as an advisor to The Alliance for Benzodiazepine Best Practices and The Council for Sustainable Healing, you can find Jocelyn rocking out to big band music and forcing her kids to watch MGM musicals with her.

www.ingramcontent.com/pod-product-compliance
Lightning Source LLC
Chambersburg PA
CBHW060321030426
42336CB00011B/1158